Oriental express

Weight Watchers ProPoints Plan

Nicola Graimes

SIMON & SCHUSTER ILLUSTRATED

London · New York · Sydney · Toronto

A CBS COMPANY

Enjoy the exotic tastes of the Far East with *Oriental Express*, the latest cookbook from the Weight Watchers range to accompany the new ***ProPoints*** plan. Now you can easily recreate the aromas and flavours of distant lands right in your own kitchen with these 60 easy-to-follow recipes. Designed with you in mind, they're not only delicious but they'll also help you make the most of your ***ProPoints*** budget.

Whether you're cooking for one or two, a family or a whole supper party, *Oriental Express* shows you how to cook traditional Far Eastern food in a way that fits with your weight loss efforts. The recipes range from rice and noodle-based ones, to wok fried dishes, to one pot meals; all based on authentic recipes from the Orient. Many of the recipes contain **Filling & Healthy Foods**, helping to keep you satisfied as you lose weight.

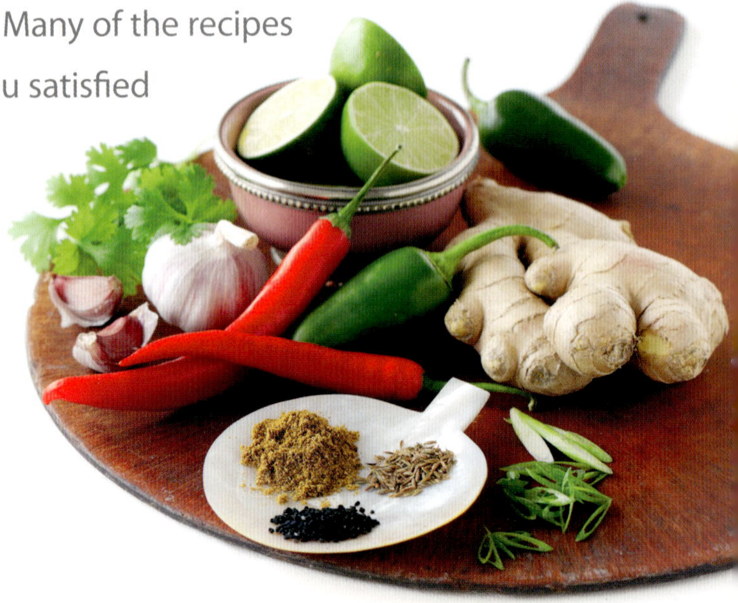

discover fabulous dishes from the Far East...

Thai burgers on page 9

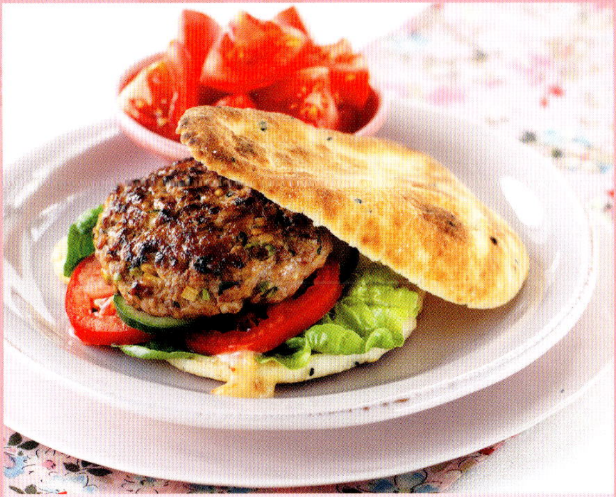

light bites
and sides

These recipes are ideal for when you simply want something light or a really tasty idea to jazz up mealtimes. Why not try a spicy snack or some delicious samosas? You'll love their fantastic oriental flavours.

***ProPoints* values per serving** 2
***ProPoints* values per recipe** 10
5 mins prep, 45 mins cooking

V **Serves 4**

410 g can **chick peas**, drained and rinsed
1 tablespoon tandoori spice mix
½ teaspoon turmeric
1 teaspoon dried chilli flakes
low fat cooking spray
salt

Roasted spiced chick peas

2 *ProPoints* value

These tasty little nibbles make a great low ***ProPoints*** value alternative to crisps and nuts and are very simple to make.

1. Preheat the oven to Gas Mark 7/220°C/fan oven 200°C.
2. Tip the chick peas into a mixing bowl and add the tandoori spice mix, turmeric and chilli flakes. Stir the chick peas until coated in the spices.
3. Spray a large non stick baking tray with the cooking spray. Tip the chick peas on to the tray and spread them out in a single layer.
4. Roast the chick peas in the oven for 40–45 minutes until crisp and golden. Remove them from the oven and transfer to a serving bowl. Season with salt before serving.

V **Variation** Instead of the tandoori spice mix, you could use tikka spice mix, garam masala or korma spice mix, for the same ***ProPoints*** values per serving.

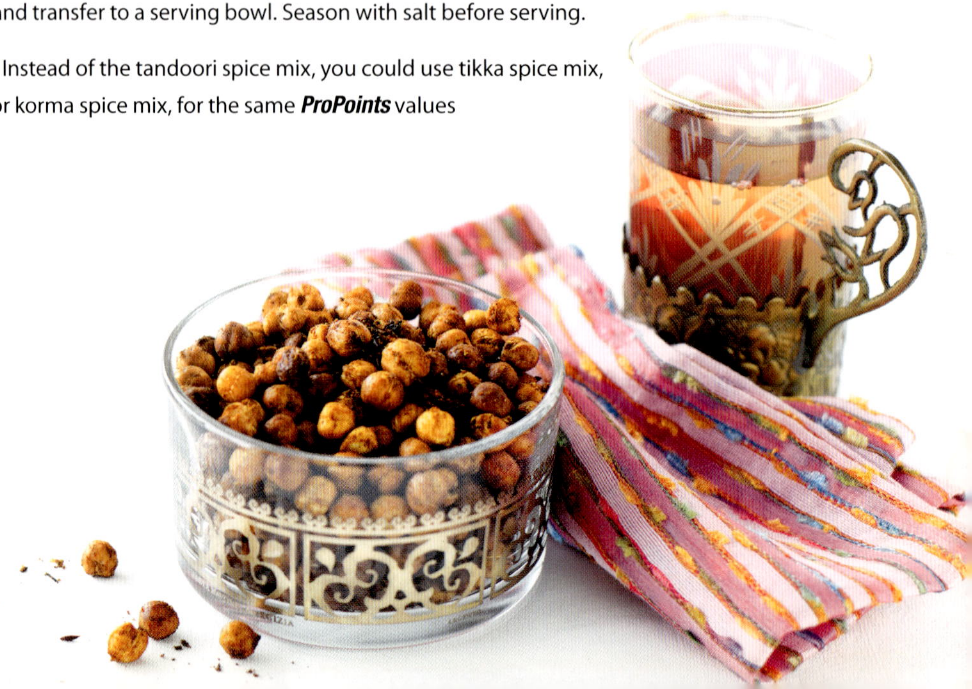

Chicken & vegetable samosas

***ProPoints* values per serving 2**
***ProPoints* values per recipe 37**
35 mins prep, 25 mins cooking

Makes 15

100 g (3½ oz) **potatoes**, such as Maris Piper, peeled and quartered
50 g (1¾ oz) frozen **petit pois**
175 g (6 oz) **skinless boneless chicken breast**, cut into bite size pieces
low fat cooking spray
1 small **onion**, chopped finely
1 small **carrot**, peeled and chopped finely
1 cm (½ inch) **fresh root ginger**, chopped finely
1 teaspoon garam masala
½ teaspoon chilli powder
½ teaspoon cumin powder
1 tablespoon lemon juice
2 tablespoons chopped **fresh coriander**
9 x 45 g (1½ oz) sheets filo pastry, measuring 50 x 24 cm (20 x 9½ inches), defrosted if frozen
salt and freshly ground black pepper

2 *ProPoints* value

Enjoy as a party nibble with 1 tablespoon of mango chutney each for 2 extra ***ProPoints*** values per serving.

1 Bring a pan of water to the boil, add the potatoes and cook for about 10 minutes or until tender. Add the peas 2 minutes before the end of the cooking time. Drain and set aside.

2 Meanwhile, heat a wok or non stick frying pan until hot. Spray the chicken with the cooking spray and stir fry for 6–8 minutes until golden and cooked through. Remove from the pan and set aside. Add the onion, carrot and ginger. Spray the vegetables with the cooking spray. Stir fry for 5 minutes, adding a splash of water if they start to stick. Stir in the spices and then transfer the mixture to a mixing bowl.

3 Cut the potatoes and chicken into small pieces and add both to the bowl with the vegetables, adding the lemon juice, coriander and seasoning.

4 Preheat the oven to Gas Mark 6/200°C/fan oven 180°C. Take three sheets of filo and place one on top of the other (keep the remaining filo covered) and then using a cutter or bowl as a template, cut out 5 x 13 cm (5 inch) rounds. Spray each round with the cooking spray and then place one round on top of the other again. Place a heaped tablespoonful of the chicken mixture on one quarter of the filo round, wet the edge with water, then fold the pastry over to make a semi-circle. Fold over again to make a triangle and pinch to seal.

5 Repeat with the remaining filo and filling to make 15 samosas. Spray two large baking trays with the cooking spray, place the samosas on top and spray again. Bake for 25 minutes until light golden. Serve warm.

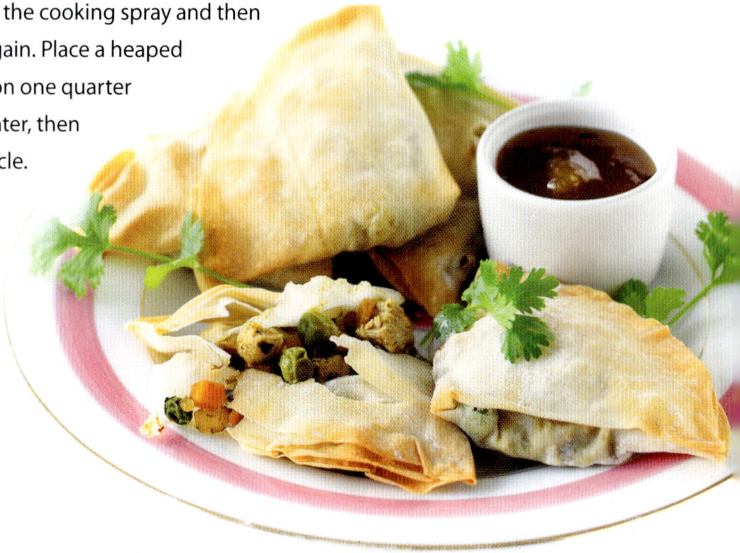

ProPoints values per serving 6
ProPoints values per recipe 11
10 mins prep + 1 hr marinating,
20 mins cooking
Serves 2

- 2 tablespoons hoisin sauce
- 1 tablespoon dark soy sauce
- 1 tablespoon clear honey
- 250 g (9 oz) **pork tenderloin**, visible fat removed
- 6 large **Little Gem lettuce leaves**
- 2.5 cm (1 inch) **cucumber**, quartered, de-seeded and cut into strips
- 1 **spring onion**, shredded
- 1 red **chilli**, de-seeded and cut into fine strips
- 6 large **fresh basil leaves**, to garnish

Pork & chilli cups

Char sui pork is a popular dish in Chinese restaurants. All you need to make it at home is a handful of store cupboard ingredients to give the pork a characteristic golden glazed coating.

1 Mix together the hoisin sauce, soy sauce and honey in a shallow dish. Add the pork and turn to coat it in the marinade. Cover and leave to marinate in the fridge for 1 hour. Preheat the oven to Gas Mark 7/220°C/fan oven 200°C.

2 Remove the pork from the dish, reserving any leftover marinade. Loosely wrap the pork in foil and place it in a roasting tray. Roast the pork for 15 minutes then remove it from the oven. If you have a combined oven and grill, turn the setting to grill and heat to medium high. If you have a separate grill, heat to the same heat.

3 Carefully remove the foil parcel from the tray, unwrap the pork and pour the cooking juices into a jug. Return it to the roasting tray, and spoon over some of the reserved marinade. Grill for 5 minutes, turning once, until golden and glossy. Slice the pork into strips.

4 Arrange the lettuce leaves on a serving plate and divide the pork between them. Top the pork with the cucumber, spring onion and chilli. Spoon over a little of the cooking juices. Garnish with basil and serve.

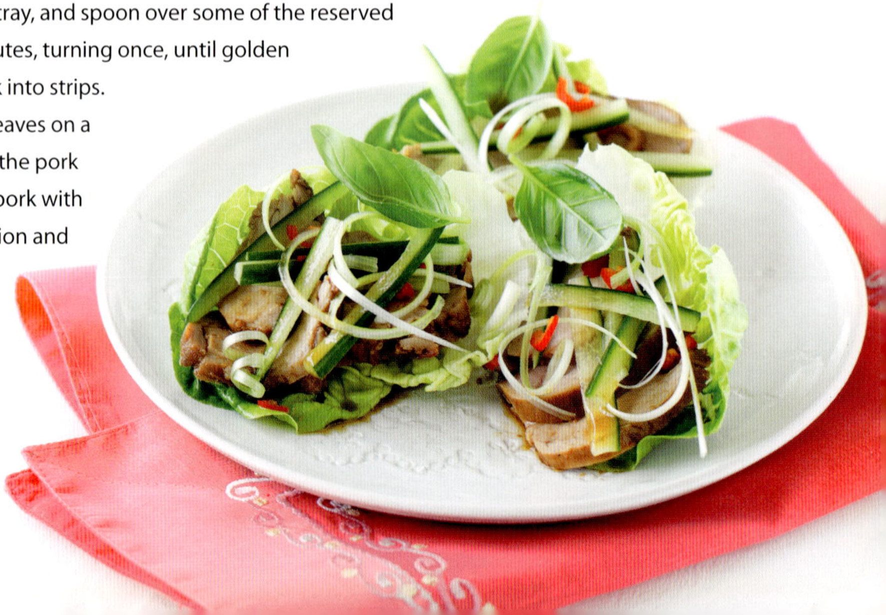

Asian beef salad

5 *ProPoints* value

ProPoints values per recipe 5
Takes 20 mins

Serves 1

125 g (4½ oz) **lean sirloin steak**, visible fat removed
low fat cooking spray
4 **Little Gem lettuce leaves**
a handful of **rocket leaves**
5 cm (2 inches) **cucumber**, halved, de-seeded and cut into ribbons
¼ small red **onion**, sliced finely
3 **cherry tomatoes**, halved
a few **fresh basil leaves**
freshly ground black pepper

For the dressing

juice of ½ a lime
½ teaspoon sugar
1 tablespoon Thai fish sauce
1 tablespoon light soy sauce
½ red **chilli**, de-seeded and chopped finely

This recipe is also ideal for any leftovers from the Sunday roast – simply follow the recipe from step 2.

1 Heat a griddle pan or the grill until very hot. Spray the steak with the cooking spray then season with black pepper. Cook the steak for 3–4 minutes, turning once, or until cooked to your liking. Leave to rest for 10 minutes then slice thinly across the grain.

2 Arrange the Little Gem and rocket leaves on a plate and top with the beef. Scatter over the cucumber, red onion and tomatoes.

3 To make the dressing, mix the lime juice with the sugar and stir until dissolved. Stir in the fish sauce, soy sauce and chilli. Pour the dressing over the salad. Season with black pepper and scatter over the basil leaves.

Variation Instead of beef, try 165 g (5¾ oz) **skinless boneless chicken breast** for the same *ProPoints* values per serving.

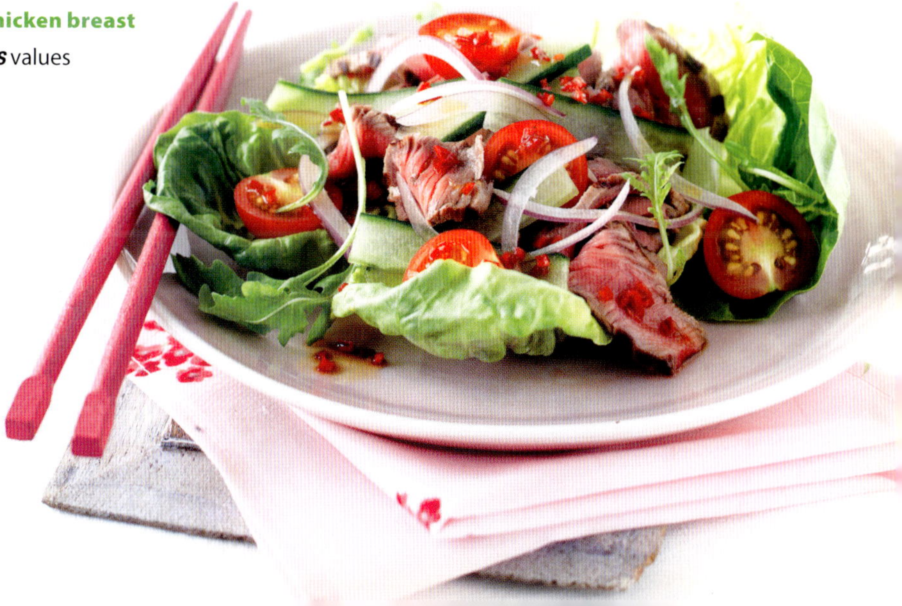

***ProPoints* values per serving** 3
***ProPoints* values per recipe** 14
10 mins prep, 55 mins cooking

V **Serves 4**

- 500 g (1 lb 2 oz) potatoes, unpeeled, scrubbed, halved lengthways and cut into wedges
- low fat cooking spray
- 2 teaspoons tikka spice mix
- salt and freshly ground black pepper

For the mint raita

- 125 g (4½ oz) low fat plain yogurt
- 5 tablespoons chopped fresh mint
- ½ teaspoon cumin seeds
- ¼ teaspoon dried chilli flakes

Tikka potato wedges

3 *ProPoints* value

These potato wedges have a light, spicy coating and are delicious served with mint raita.

1 Preheat the oven to Gas Mark 7/220°C/fan oven 200°C. Pat dry the potatoes with kitchen towel then put them in a mixing bowl. Spray with the cooking spray, stirring the potatoes as you do. Sprinkle with the tikka spice mix, season and stir the potatoes again to coat them in the spices.

2 Spray a large non stick baking tray with the cooking spray and arrange the potatoes on the tray. Bake for about 50–55 minutes, turning twice, until golden.

3 While the potatoes are roasting, make the mint raita by mixing together the yogurt and mint in a small bowl. Season and stir until combined then sprinkle with the cumin seeds and dried chilli flakes. Serve with the potato wedges.

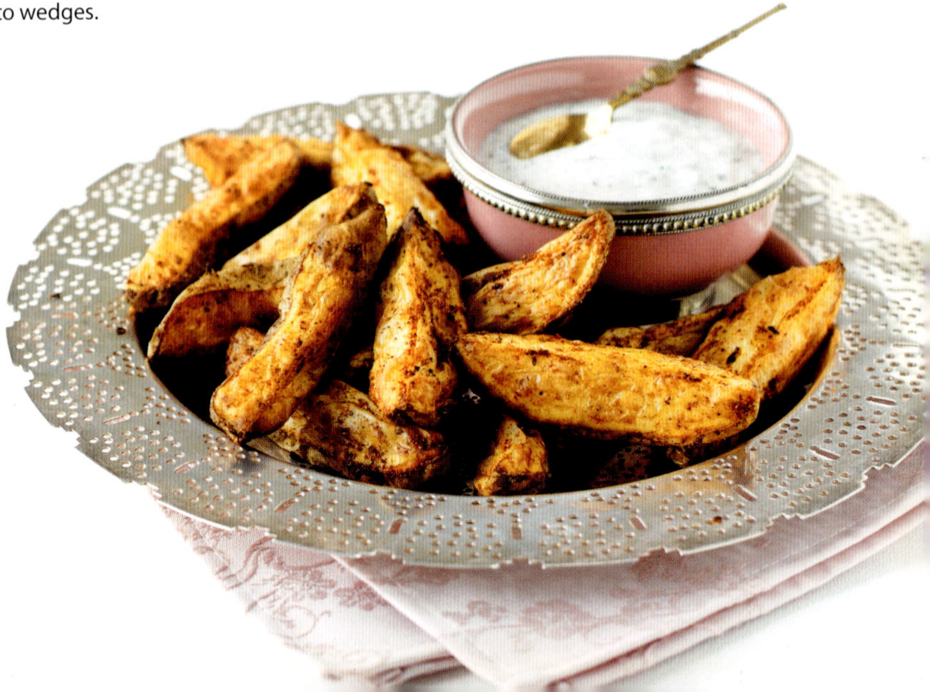

ProPoints values per serving 9
ProPoints values per recipe 38
Takes 25 mins + 30 mins chilling

Serves 4

500 g (1 lb 2 oz) lean turkey mince
4 spring onions, chopped finely
3 large garlic cloves, crushed
4 teaspoons Thai red curry paste
3 tablespoons chopped fresh coriander
low fat cooking spray
salt and freshly ground black pepper

To serve

1 tablespoon extra light mayonnaise
2 tablespoons sweet chilli sauce
2 teaspoons lime juice
4 plain mini naan breads
4 Little Gem lettuce leaves
8 cucumber slices
8 tomato slices

Thai burgers

9 *ProPoints* value

These spicy burgers make a great light meal.

1 Mix together the turkey mince, spring onions, garlic, curry paste and coriander in a bowl then season. Using your hands, form the turkey mixture into four burgers then chill, covered, for 30 minutes.

2 Spray a non stick frying pan with the cooking spray and fry the burgers for 5 minutes on each side or until cooked through and golden. Preheat the grill to medium high.

3 Meanwhile, mix together the mayonnaise, chilli sauce and lime juice. Warm the naan under the grill for 2 minutes, turning once, then split open. Spread the inside of each naan with the mayonnaise mixture then top each with a lettuce leaf, two slices of cucumber, two slices of tomato and a burger. Serve immediately.

V **Variation** You can replace the turkey mince with 250 g (9 oz) tofu, drained and grated coarsely, and follow the recipe from step 1. The *ProPoints* values will be 7 per serving.

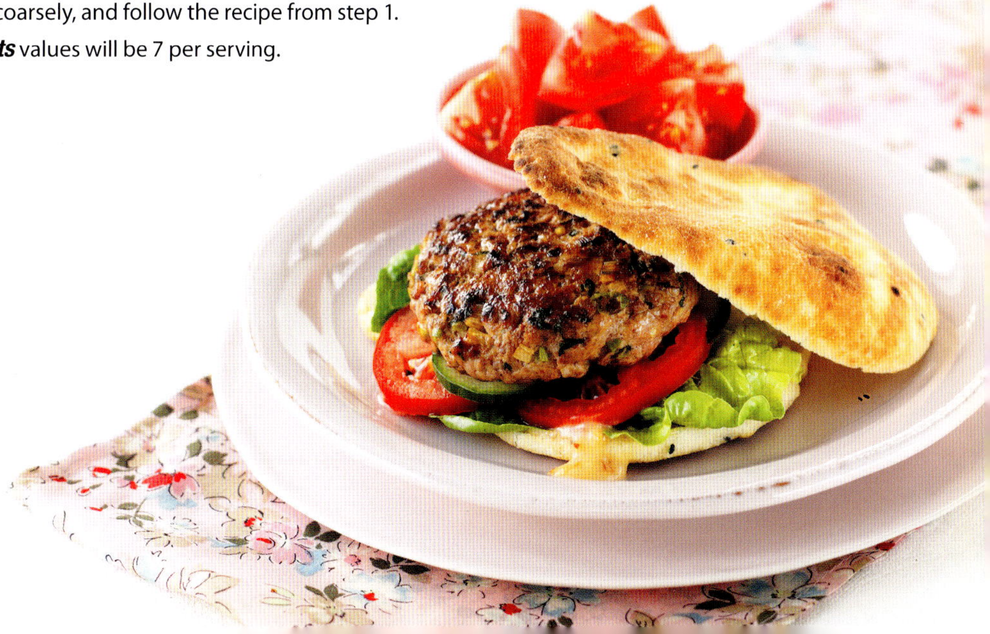

***ProPoints* values per serving** 7
***ProPoints* values per recipe** 36
Takes 50 mins

Makes 5

200 g (7 oz) plain flour, plus 5 tablespoons for dusting
½ teaspoon salt
1 tablespoon vegetable oil
low fat cooking spray
100 g (3½ oz) potatoes, peeled and quartered
1 small onion, chopped finely
1 teaspoon black mustard seeds
½ teaspoon ground turmeric

Stuffed paratha

7 *ProPoints* value

Enjoy with 1 tablespoon per person of the mint raita on page 8 for an extra 1 ***ProPoints*** value per serving.

1 Sift the flour and salt into a mixing bowl, stir and then make a well in the centre. Pour in 125 ml (4 fl oz) tepid water and the oil. Stir with a fork until combined then use your hands to form the mixture into a soft ball of dough. It should be fairly sticky so add more water if the dough is too dry.

2 Lightly dust a clean work surface with 3 tablespoons of the flour and knead the dough for 5 minutes until it becomes smooth. Spray a clean bowl with the cooking spray, add the dough, spray the dough again, cover and set aside for 30 minutes. Meanwhile, bring a pan of water to the boil, add the potatoes and cook until tender. Drain then mash. Leave to cool.

3 Heat a non stick frying pan until hot, spray with the cooking spray and fry the onion for 4 minutes then add the mustard seeds and continue to cook for another 2 minutes. Stir in the turmeric then transfer to a bowl with the mashed potato. Beat together to form a paste.

4 Divide the dough into five pieces. Lightly dust a work surface with the remaining 2 tablespoons of flour. Roll each piece of dough into a circle, about 19 cm (7½ inches) in diameter and 1 cm (½ inch) thick. Spread 2 teaspoons of the potato mixture over one half of the dough then fold into a semi-circle, and then fold again into quarters. Roll out until about 19 cm (7½ inches) in diameter (the shape doesn't need to be round). Pat off any excess flour.

5 Heat a large non stick frying pan until hot. Spray with the cooking spray and cook the breads, one at a time, for 2 minutes on each side until light golden. They are best served warm.

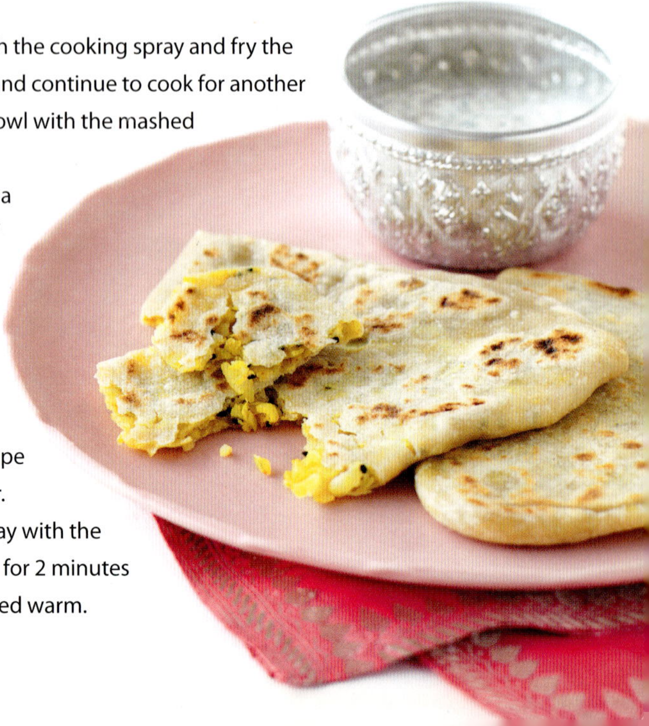

ProPoints **values per serving 7**
ProPoints **values per recipe 14**
Takes 40 mins

Serves 2

85 g (3 oz) dried sushi rice
2 tablespoons rice vinegar
½ teaspoon caster sugar
¼ teaspoon salt
1½ x 2½ g nori sheets
1 tablespoon extra light mayonnaise
1 heaped teaspoon wasabi paste
75 g (2¾ oz) cooked **smoked trout** or **salmon**, broken into large flakes
6 **watercress** sprigs, tough stalks removed
6 thin **cucumber** sticks (about 5 cm/2 inches long), de-seeded

To serve

4 tablespoons light soy sauce
25 g (1 oz) pickled ginger

Simple sushi cones

7 *ProPoints* value

These elegant nori and smoked fish cones really are very easy to make.

1 Put the rice in a lidded saucepan and add 150 ml (5 fl oz) water. Bring to the boil, then reduce the heat to its lowest setting, cover and simmer for 12–15 minutes until the water is absorbed and the grains are tender. Set aside for 5 minutes, covered.

2 Meanwhile, mix together the rice vinegar, sugar and salt. Put the rice in a mixing bowl then gently stir in the rice vinegar mixture and leave to cool for about 30 minutes.

3 Cut the nori sheets into 10 cm (4 inch) squares for a total of six squares. Mix together the mayonnaise and wasabi then smear over the dull side of each nori square. Using wet hands, place 2 teaspoons of rice diagonally across each square then top with a few flakes of trout or salmon, a sprig of watercress and a cucumber stick.

4 Wet one edge of the nori and roll into a cone shape. Press the edge to seal. Repeat to make a total of six cones. Serve three cones each, with small bowls of soy sauce and the pickled ginger.

Cook's tip Seal the package of nori sheets and they'll keep well in the cupboard, ready for the next time you decide to make this recipe.

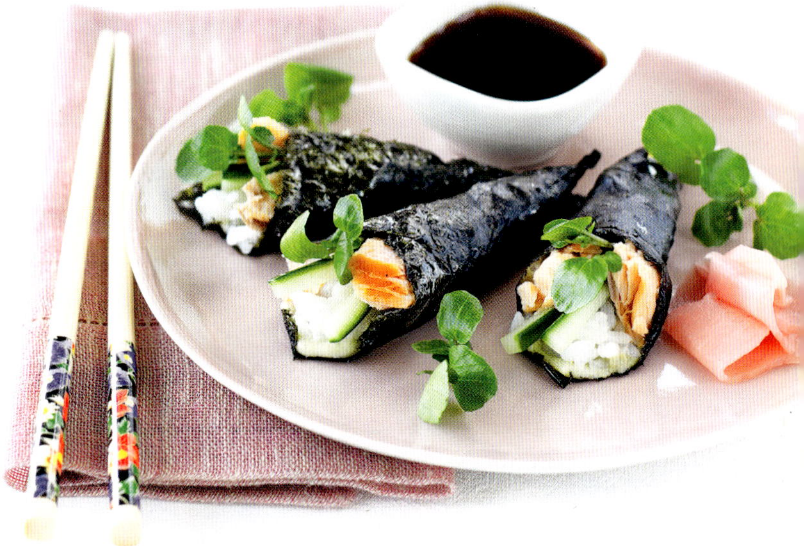

ProPoints **values per serving 3**
ProPoints **values per recipe 6**
Takes 15 mins

V Serves 2

- low fat cooking spray
- 2 large **spring onions**, chopped finely
- 1 small red **pepper,** de-seeded and diced
- ½ stalk **lemongrass**, peeled and chopped finely
- 1 cm (½ inch) **fresh root ginger**, chopped finely
- 3 **eggs**, lightly beaten
- 1 teaspoon light soy sauce
- freshly ground black pepper

Oriental scrambled eggs

3 *ProPoints* value

Serve with a warm, plain mini naan bread each for an extra 3 ***ProPoints*** values per serving.

1 Heat a wok or non stick frying pan until hot, and spray with the cooking spray. Add the spring onions, pepper, lemongrass and ginger, then stir fry for 1 minute.

2 Season the eggs with black pepper and pour them into the pan. Using a spatula, gently stir and turn the eggs until they scramble, scraping the bottom of the pan to prevent the eggs from sticking; this should take 2–3 minutes. Gently stir in the soy sauce. Serve immediately.

Cook's tip For successful scrambled eggs, it's important to use a heavy based, non stick saucepan or frying pan.

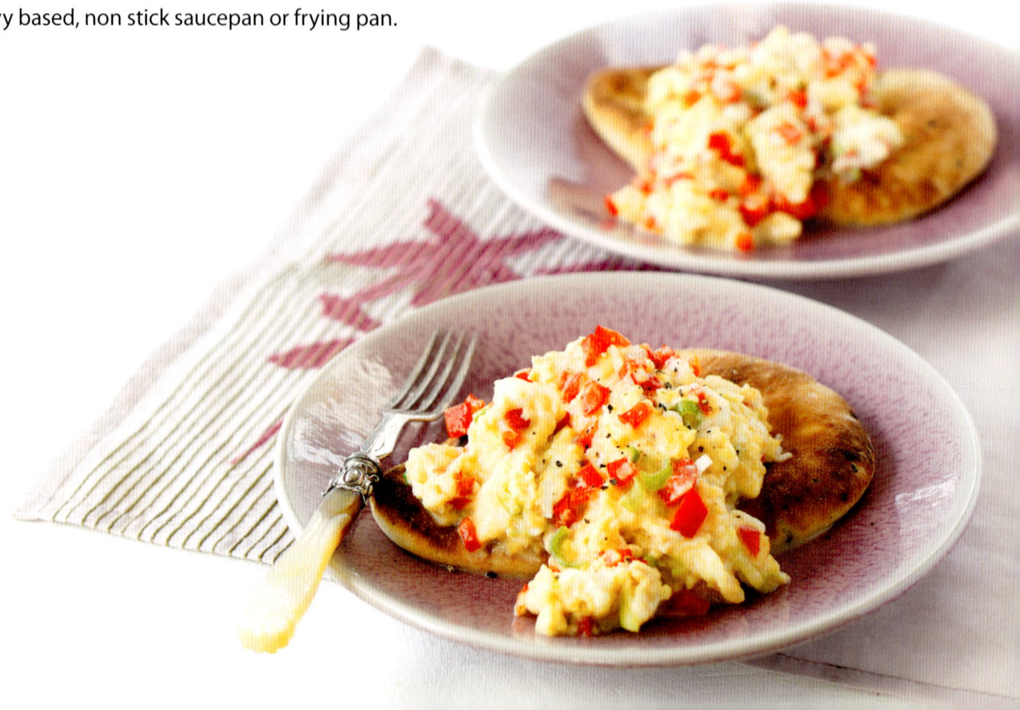

rice
and noodles

Tuck into some of your favourite rice and noodle classics and enjoy substantial meals with sensational flavours any time of the week. The Nasi Goreng and Easy Spiced Lamb are ideal as midweek meals.

Chicken chow mein on page 20

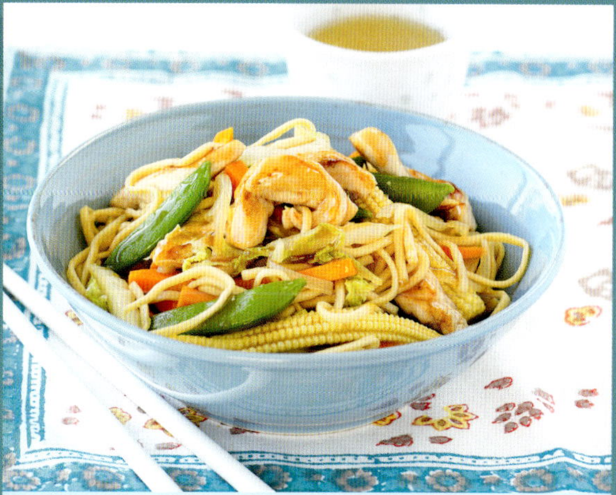

ProPoints values per serving 7
ProPoints values per recipe 28
Takes 35 mins

rice mixture only — **Serves 4**

- 200 g (7 oz) dried **brown basmati rice**, rinsed
- 1 **pineapple**, halved lengthways, green leaves trimmed, if necessary
- low fat cooking spray
- 1 large **onion**, diced
- 2 large **garlic cloves**, chopped finely
- 2.5 cm (1 inch) **fresh root ginger**, chopped finely
- 1 teaspoon Chinese five spice
- 100 g (3½ oz) frozen **petit pois**
- 175 g (6 oz) thick cut **premium ham**, visible fat removed, diced
- 1 red **chilli**, de-seeded and chopped finely (optional)
- 2 tablespoons light soy sauce
- freshly ground black pepper
- 2 tablespoons chopped **fresh coriander**, to garnish

Chinese rice with pineapple & ham

7 ProPoints value

1 Put the rice in a lidded saucepan and cover with 450 ml (16 fl oz) water. Bring to the boil, then reduce the heat to its lowest setting. Cover and simmer for 25 minutes until the water is absorbed and the grains are tender. Set aside for 5 minutes, covered, then spread out on a large plate to cool.

2 Meanwhile, to hollow out the pineapple shells, cut the fruit vertically then slice away the flesh to leave two hollow shells. Slice the hard core off the flesh and cut the fruit into bite size pieces – you want about 200 g (7 oz) pineapple. Set aside any remaining fruit for later use.

3 Heat a large wok or non stick frying pan until hot. Spray with the cooking spray then stir fry the onion over a medium heat for 3 minutes. Add the garlic, ginger, Chinese five spice, petit pois, ham, chilli, if using, and pineapple. Stir fry for 1 minute then add the rice, soy sauce and a splash of water. Stir everything until combined and heated through.

4 Season with black pepper, spoon into the pineapple shells and garnish with fresh coriander.

Variations You could use 200 g (7 oz) canned **pineapple in natural juice**, drained, instead of the fresh fruit. If using fresh pineapple, you can use the leftover fruit to make the Pineapple and Ginger Sorbet on page 60.

V Omit the ham and stir in two beaten **eggs** while you are adding the rice in step 3. Stir the rice over a medium heat until the egg is cooked; this should take about 2–3 minutes. The ***ProPoints*** values per serving will remain the same.

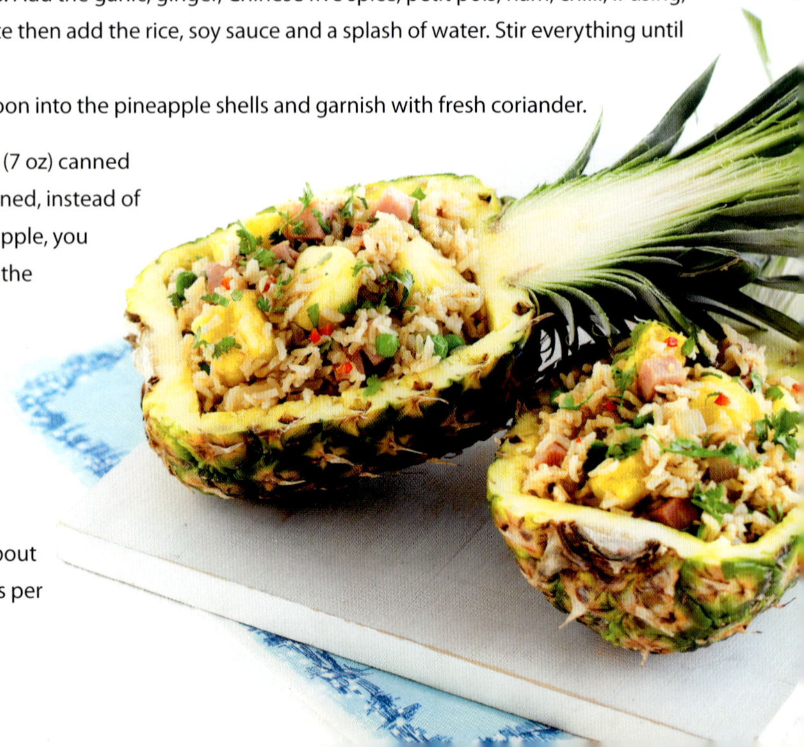

ProPoints values per serving 10
ProPoints values per recipe 41
Takes 40 mins

Serves 4

200 g (7 oz) dried **brown basmati rice**, rinsed
125 g (4½ oz) fine **green beans**, trimmed
125 g (4½ oz) small **cauliflower** florets
low fat cooking spray
1 **onion**, chopped
3 large **garlic cloves**, chopped
2.5 cm (1 inch) **fresh root ginger**, chopped finely
1 large **courgette**, diced
350 g (12 oz) lean diced lamb, visible fat removed
50 g (1¾ oz) dried apricots, chopped into small pieces
2 tablespoons garam masala
½ teaspoon chilli powder
salt and freshly ground black pepper

Easy spiced lamb

10 *ProPoints* value

1 Put the rice in a lidded saucepan and cover with 450 ml (16 fl oz) water. Bring to the boil, then reduce the heat to its lowest setting, cover, and simmer for 25 minutes until the water is absorbed and the grains are tender. Set aside for 5 minutes, covered, then remove the lid and leave to cool slightly.

2 Bring about 2.5 cm (1 inch) of water to the boil in a lidded pan. Put the green beans and cauliflower in a steamer basket and place it over the pan. Cover and cook for 5 minutes until al dente (they shouldn't be completely cooked). Alternatively, bring a small amount of water to the boil and cook the vegetables for 5 minutes then drain. Refresh under cold running water then set aside.

3 Heat a large lidded wok or non stick frying pan. Spray with the cooking spray and stir fry the onion over a medium heat for 4 minutes. Add the garlic, ginger and courgette and stir fry for 3 minutes. Next, add the lamb and stir fry for a further 3 minutes until browned.

4 Add the apricots and spices, stir, and then add the green beans, cauliflower, rice and 5 tablespoons of water. Stir until combined and then cover with a lid and heat through for 5 minutes. Season before serving.

Variation You can replace the lamb with four hard boiled **eggs** for 8 ***ProPoints*** values per serving. Halve the eggs and place on top of the cooked rice just before serving.

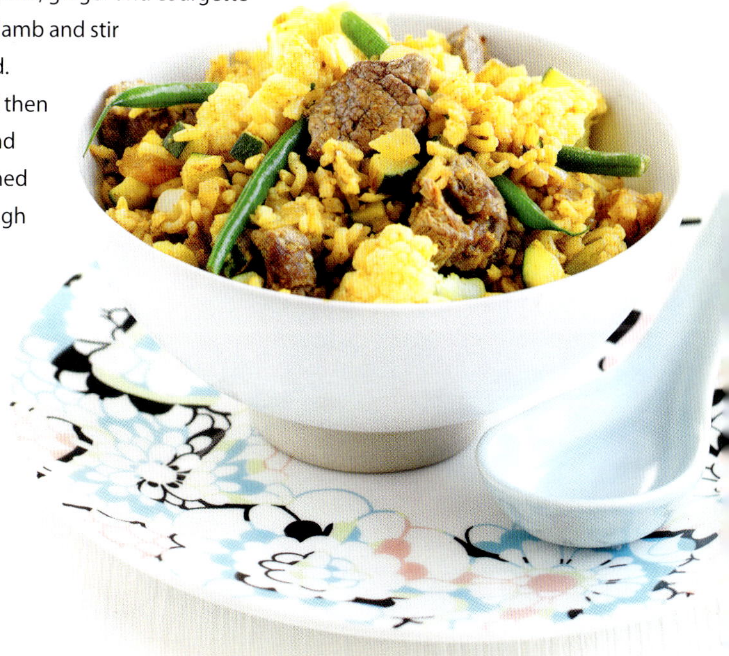

Nasi goreng

***ProPoints* values per recipe** **8**
Takes 20 mins

Serves 1

- 50 g (1¾ oz) dried long grain rice
- low fat cooking spray
- 2 **shallots**, diced
- 50 g (1¾ oz) button **mushrooms**, sliced
- 1 red **chilli**, de-seeded and chopped
- 1 small **carrot**, quartered and sliced
- 75 g (2¾ oz) white **cabbage**, shredded
- 1 cm (½ inch) **fresh root ginger**, chopped finely
- 100 g (3½ oz) cooked **prawns**
- 1 tablespoon tomato ketchup
- 1 tablespoon light soy sauce
- freshly ground black pepper
- a few **watercress** sprigs, to garnish

This popular Indonesian dish is ideal for using up any leftover cooked rice. For the best results, make sure the cooked rice is cold then reheat it until piping hot.

1. Bring a pan of water to the boil, add the rice and cook according to the packet instructions until tender. Heat a wok or non stick frying pan until hot. Spray with the cooking spray and stir fry the shallots over a medium heat for 2 minutes.
2. Add the mushrooms, chilli, carrot, cabbage and ginger, spray again with the cooking spray, and stir fry for 3–4 minutes, adding a splash of water if they start to stick.
3. Stir in the rice, prawns, ketchup and soy sauce and stir until combined and heated through. Season with black pepper and serve garnished with watercress.

V Variation Replace the prawns with 75 g (2¾ oz) marinated **tofu** pieces. Add the tofu in step 2 with the vegetables. The ***ProPoints*** values will be the same.

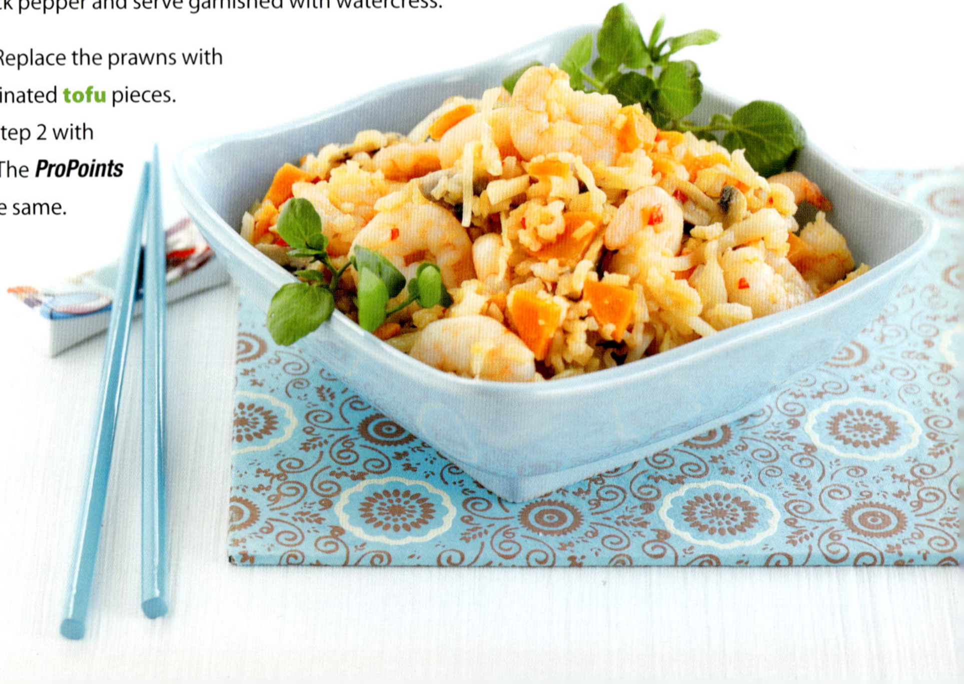

***ProPoints* values per serving** 11
Takes 25 mins + 1 hr marinating

Serves 1

- 1 teaspoon sweet chilli sauce
- 1 tablespoon dark soy sauce
- 1 tablespoon mirin
- 125 g (4½ oz) **lean pork loin steak**, visible fat removed
- low fat cooking spray
- 40 g (1½ oz) dried rice noodles
- 2 chestnut **mushrooms**, sliced
- 1 small **carrot**, peeled and cut into matchsticks
- 1 cm (½ inch) **fresh root ginger**, cut into matchsticks
- 40 g (1½ oz) baby **spinach leaves**
- 1 sachet (18 g) miso paste
- 25 g (1 oz) **beansprouts**
- 1 **spring onion**, sliced diagonally
- ¼ teaspoon dried chilli flakes (optional)

Chilli pork ramen

11 *ProPoints* value

1 Mix together the chilli sauce, soy sauce and mirin in a shallow dish. Add the pork, spoon over the marinade and leave to marinate for 1 hour.

2 Heat a non stick frying pan until hot. Remove the pork from the marinade (reserving the marinade), put in the pan and spray with the cooking spray. Cook for 2–3 minutes on each side, depending on the thickness of the pork, until browned and cooked through. Remove from the pan, cover with foil and set aside.

3 Meanwhile, bring a pan of water to the boil and cook the noodles according to the packet instructions, then drain and rinse under cold running water. Place in a bowl, cover with cold water, and set aside.

4 Put the mushrooms, carrot, ginger, spinach and reserved marinade in a lidded saucepan, add 200 ml (7 fl oz) water, stir and bring to the boil. Reduce the heat, stir in the miso paste then simmer, partially covered, for 2 minutes until the vegetables are just tender.

5 Drain the noodles and put them in a large shallow bowl. Pour over the vegetable soup. Slice the pork on the diagonal and arrange on top of the soup. Sprinkle with the beansprouts, spring onion and chilli flakes, if using. Serve immediately.

V Variation You can replace the pork with the same amount of Japanese soft **tofu**. Cut into cubes and place on top of the soup in step 5 before adding the garnishes. The ***ProPoints*** values will be 10.

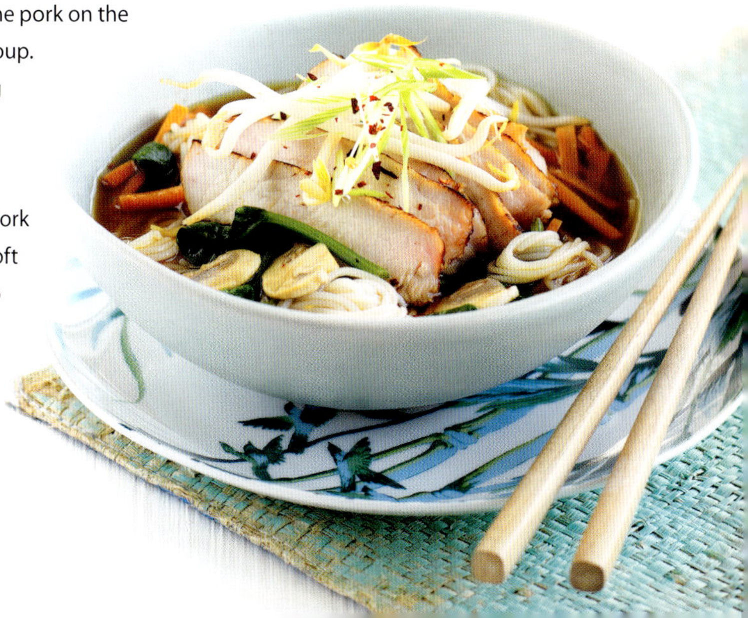

***ProPoints* values per serving**	**10**
***ProPoints* values per recipe**	**19**

15 mins prep, 25 mins cooking

Serves 2

Oriental mushroom risotto

10 *ProPoints* value

low fat cooking spray
1 **onion**, diced
1 cm (½ inch) **fresh root ginger**, chopped finely
100 g (3½ oz) chestnut **mushrooms**, quartered
100 g (3½ oz) shiitake **mushrooms**, stalks removed, sliced
150 g (5½ oz) dried risotto rice
6 tablespoons Chinese cooking wine or dry sherry
600 ml (20 fl oz) vegetable stock
1 tablespoon light soy sauce
2 tablespoons chopped **fresh coriander**
freshly ground black pepper

Serve with steamed fine **green beans** for no extra ***ProPoints*** values.

1 Spray a medium size lidded saucepan with the cooking spray. Add the onion, cover and cook over a medium heat for 5 minutes, stirring occasionally until softened. Add the ginger, mushrooms, and rice, spray again with the cooking spray and cook for 1 minute, stirring, until the rice is opaque. Add a splash of water if it is very dry.

2 Pour in the Chinese wine or sherry and cook for about 2 minutes until reduced. Turn down the heat to low and then add a ladleful of stock and stir until it is absorbed. Continue to add the stock, a ladleful at a time, stirring continuously until the rice is creamy but still a little al dente. This should take about 20–25 minutes.

3 Stir in the soy sauce and half of the coriander. Season with black pepper and serve garnished with the remaining coriander.

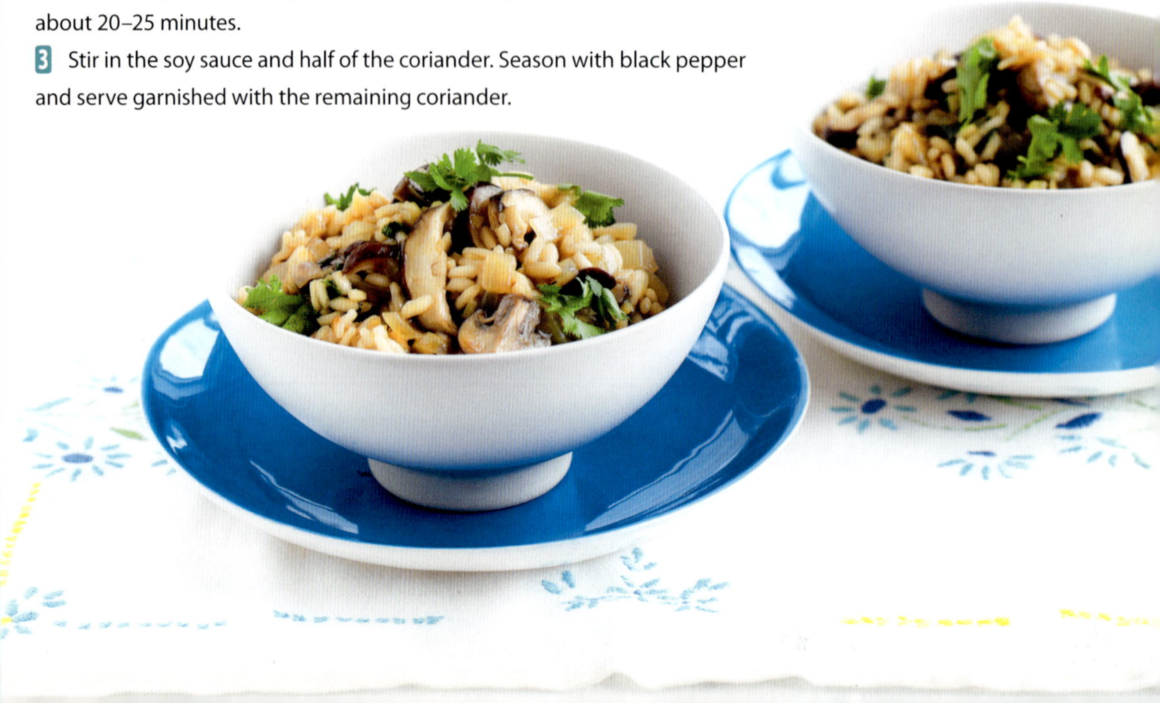

Beef yakisoba

***ProPoints* values per serving** **8**
***ProPoints* values per recipe** **33**
Takes 30 mins + 30 mins marinating

Serves 4

2 tablespoons mirin
4 tablespoons light soy sauce
1 teaspoon toasted sesame oil
350 g (12 oz) lean beef fillet, cut into strips
175 g (6 oz) dried soba noodles
low fat cooking spray
1 onion, halved and sliced thinly
125 g (4½ oz) mange tout
1 green pepper, de-seeded and sliced thinly
2.5 cm (1 inch) fresh root ginger, chopped finely
125 g (4½ oz) beansprouts
freshly ground black pepper

To garnish

2 spring onions, chopped finely
1 tablespoon pink pickled ginger
1 teaspoon sesame seeds

Soba noodles have a deliciously nutty taste and make the perfect partner for beef in this recipe.

1 Mix together the mirin, soy sauce and sesame oil in a shallow dish. Add the beef, spoon the marinade over and leave to marinate for 30 minutes.

2 Meanwhile, bring a pan of water to the boil and cook the noodles according to the packet instructions. Drain then refresh under cold running water. Place in a bowl, cover with cold water, then set aside.

3 Meanwhile, heat a large wok or non stick frying pan until hot. Remove the beef from the marinade (reserving the marinade). Add the beef to the pan and spray with the cooking spray. Stir fry for 2–3 minutes until browned all over. Transfer the beef and any juices to a bowl and set aside.

4 Add the onion, mange tout, green pepper and ginger to the pan, spray with the cooking spray and stir fry for 3 minutes, adding 1 tablespoon of water if it starts to stick. Add the beansprouts, beef, juices and reserved marinade and stir fry for another minute.

5 Drain the noodles and add them to the pan, turning them until combined and warmed through. Divide between four large shallow bowls. Season with black pepper and garnish each serving with the spring onions, pickled ginger and sesame seeds.

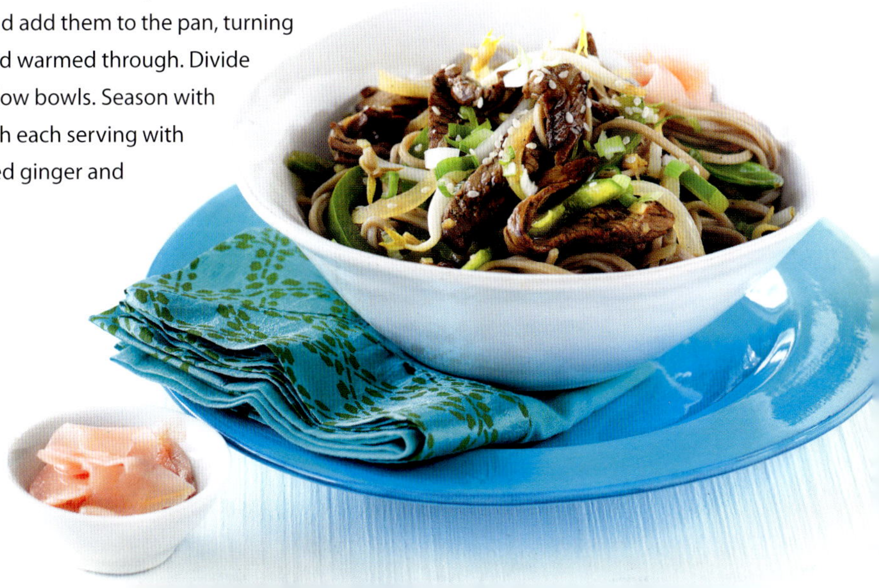

Chicken chow mein

10 ProPoints value

***ProPoints* values per serving 10**
***ProPoints* values per recipe 42**
Takes 25 mins + 30 mins marinating

Serves 4

- 600 g (1 lb 5 oz) **skinless boneless chicken breasts**, cut into strips
- 6 tablespoons soy sauce
- 200 g (7 oz) dried egg noodles
- low fat cooking spray
- 1 large **onion**, sliced
- 1 **carrot**, peeled and halved crossways and cut into batons
- 100 g (3½ oz) **baby corn**, halved lengthways
- 100 g (3½ oz) **sugar snap peas**
- 2 large **garlic cloves**, sliced thinly
- 2.5 cm (1 inch) **fresh root ginger**, chopped finely
- 150 g (5½ oz) **Chinese leaves**, sliced thinly
- 2 tablespoons Chinese cooking wine or dry sherry
- 4 tablespoons oyster sauce
- freshly ground black pepper

Chow mein simply means 'stir fried noodles'. This popular dish is very tasty and so quick to make.

1 Marinate the chicken in 4 tablespoons of soy sauce for 30 minutes. Bring a pan of water to the boil and cook the noodles according to the packet instructions, then drain and refresh under cold running water. Place in a bowl, cover with cold water, then set aside.

2 Remove the chicken from the soy sauce and discard the marinade. Heat a large wok or non stick frying pan, add the chicken, spray with the cooking spray and stir fry for 4–5 minutes until golden and cooked. Remove from the pan and set aside.

3 Add the onion, carrot, baby corn and sugar snap peas to the pan, spray with the cooking spray and stir fry for 3 minutes. Add the garlic, ginger and Chinese leaves then stir fry for another minute.

4 Drain the cooked noodles and add to the pan with the Chinese cooking wine or sherry, the remaining soy sauce, oyster sauce and chicken and stir until combined and heated through. Season with black pepper, then serve in large shallow bowls.

V Variation Replace the chicken with 150 g (5½ oz) chestnut **mushrooms**, quartered, and 150 g (5½ oz) tenderstem **broccoli** and add in step 3 with the other vegetables, for 7 ***ProPoints*** values per serving.

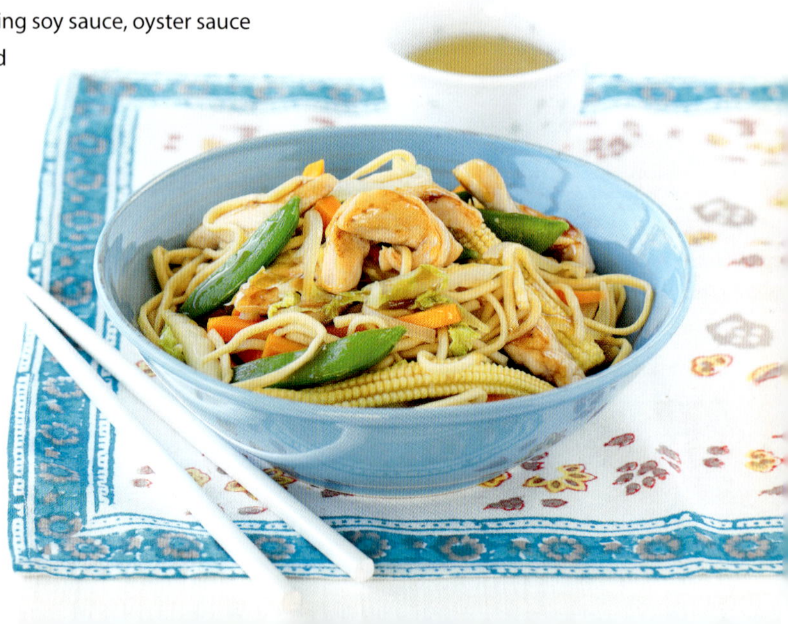

ProPoints values per serving 10
ProPoints values per recipe 21
Takes 35 mins

Serves 2

- 100 g (3½ oz) dried wholewheat noodles
- 1 teaspoon sesame seeds
- 300 g (10½ oz) **skinless boneless chicken breasts**, cut into large bite size pieces
- low fat cooking spray
- 50 g (1¾ oz) baby **spinach leaves**, long stalks discarded
- 75 g (2¾ oz) **radishes**, trimmed and sliced into rounds
- 2 **spring onions**, sliced diagonally
- 5 cm (2 inches) **cucumber**, quartered, de-seeded and cut into thin strips
- a few **fresh basil** leaves

For the dressing

- 1 cm (½ inch) **fresh root ginger**, grated
- 1 tablespoon balsamic vinegar
- 1 tablespoon light soy sauce
- 2 tablespoons fresh orange juice
- ½ teaspoon toasted sesame oil
- a pinch of dried chilli flakes (optional)

Oriental chicken noodle salad

10 *ProPoints* value

Fresh and vibrant, this substantial salad has a wonderfully flavoursome ginger, soy and orange dressing. The chilli is optional but it does give a warming lift.

1 Bring a pan of water to the boil and cook the noodles according to the packet instructions, then drain and refresh under cold running water. Place in a bowl, cover with cold water, then set aside.

2 Heat a large wok or non stick frying pan and dry fry the sesame seeds for about 3 minutes, turning occasionally, until golden. Remove from the pan and set aside.

3 Spray the chicken pieces with the cooking spray and place in the hot wok or frying pan. Stir fry for 6–8 minutes until cooked and golden all over.

4 Meanwhile, make the dressing. Squeeze the ginger, using your hands, and mix the juice with the rest of the dressing ingredients. Discard the remaining fibrous bits of ginger. Drain the noodles, return to the bowl and then combine with the spinach, radishes, spring onions and cucumber. Spoon over the dressing, toss together and then divide between two large shallow bowls or plates. Top with the chicken, basil leaves and sesame seeds. Serve hot or cold.

V Variation You can replace the chicken with 200 g (7 oz) **Quorn** pieces for 9 *ProPoints* values per serving. Add them in step 3 and stir fry for about 3 minutes until slightly golden.

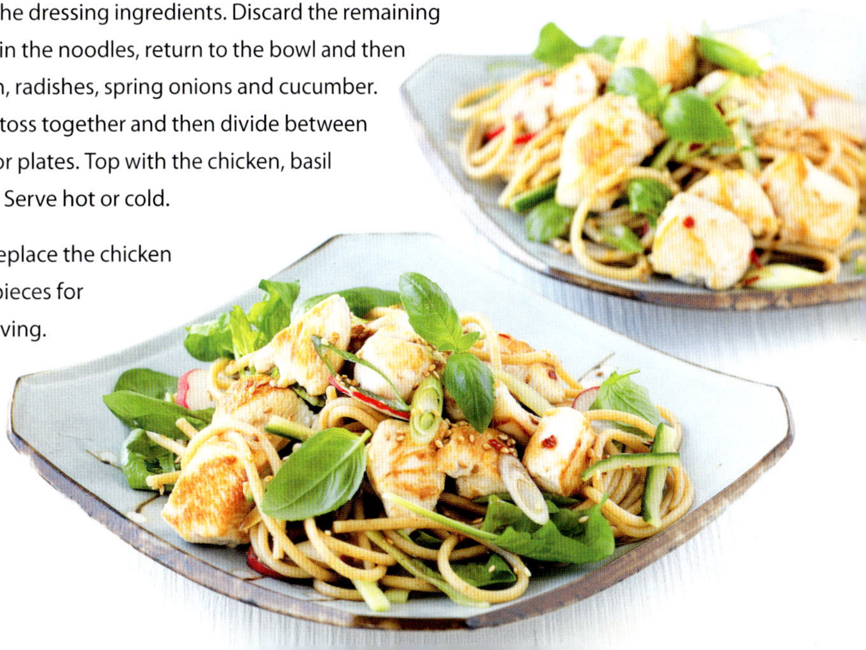

ProPoints values per serving 12
ProPoints values per recipe 23
Takes 20 mins

Serves 2

100 g (3½ oz) dried medium egg noodles
75 g (2¾ oz) frozen soya beans
1 teaspoon sunflower oil
1 red chilli, de-seeded and chopped
2 garlic cloves, chopped finely
3 spring onions, sliced diagonally
1 cm (½ inch) fresh root ginger, chopped finely
low fat cooking spray
170 g can white crab meat in brine, drained
juice of 1 large lime plus zest of ½ the lime
2 tablespoons light soy sauce
2 tablespoons chopped fresh coriander

Crab, chilli & lime noodles

12 ProPoints value

The fresh and zingy flavours of ginger, chilli and lime sing out in this speedy noodle dish. Serve with steamed pak choi for no added **ProPoints** values.

1 Bring a pan of water to the boil and cook the noodles according to the packet instructions, adding the soya beans for the last 2 minutes of cooking. Return to the boil and cook until the noodles and beans are tender. Drain, refresh under cold running water and set aside.

2 Heat the sunflower oil in a large wok or non stick frying pan. Add the chilli, garlic, spring onions and ginger and then stir fry for 30 seconds.

3 Spray the mixture with the cooking spray and add the cooked noodles, soya beans, crab, lime juice and zest, soy sauce and half of the coriander. Stir until combined and heated through. Serve sprinkled with the remaining coriander.

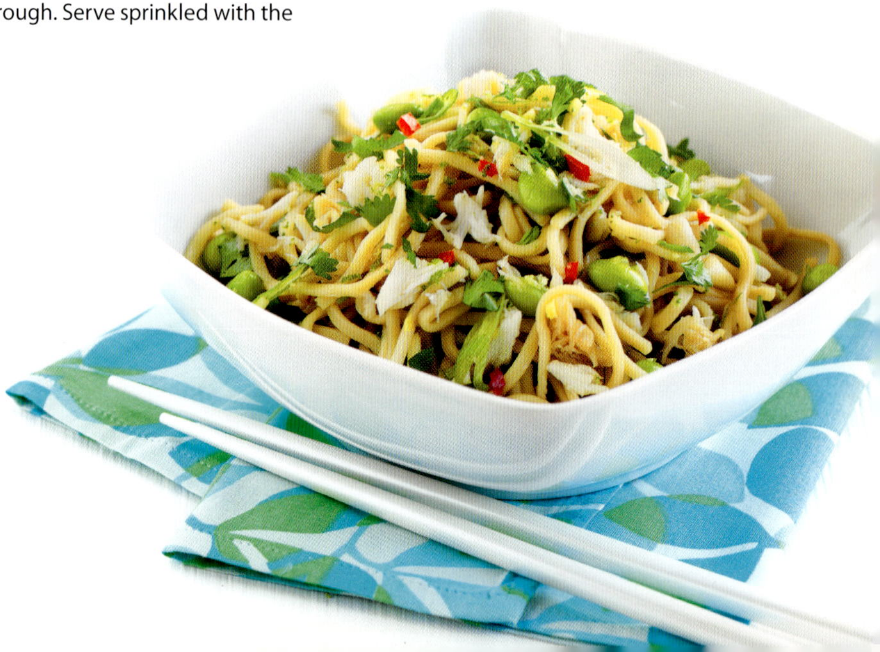

ProPoints **values per serving 8**
ProPoints **values per recipe 17**
20 mins prep, 20 mins cooking

V **Serves 2**

- low fat cooking spray
- 1 **onion**, chopped
- 2 large **garlic cloves**, chopped finely
- 60 g (2 oz) Thai red curry paste
- 300 ml (10 fl oz) vegetable stock
- 100 ml (3½ fl oz) light coconut milk
- 200 g (7 oz) **butternut squash**, peeled, de-seeded and cut into bite size pieces
- 1 small red **pepper**, de-seeded and cut into bite size pieces
- 100 g (3½ oz) chestnut **mushrooms**, quartered
- ½ teaspoon dried chilli flakes
- 1 tablespoon unsalted peanuts
- ½ teaspoon fructose or caster sugar
- 1 tablespoon lime juice
- a small handful of **fresh basil leaves**
- 200 g (7 oz) straight-to-wok udon noodles
- salt and freshly ground black pepper

Chiang Mai noodles

This vegetable and noodle one pot meal makes use of ready prepared Thai red curry paste to create a delicious, richly flavoured sauce.

1. Heat a lidded saucepan to a high heat, spray with the cooking spray and add the onion. Stir fry for 5 minutes until softened, adding a splash of water if the onions start to stick. Add the garlic then the curry paste and cook, stirring, for 1 minute.
2. Pour in the stock and coconut milk. Bring to the boil then reduce the heat and simmer, partially covered, for 4 minutes. Add the squash, red pepper, mushrooms and chilli flakes, stir then simmer, partially covered, for 20 minutes until tender.
3. Meanwhile, put the peanuts in a dry frying pan and dry fry for about 3 minutes until they smell lightly toasted. Remove from the pan then chop roughly.
4. Stir the fructose or sugar, lime juice, basil leaves and noodles into the saucepan and gently heat through. Season and serve sprinkled with the peanuts.

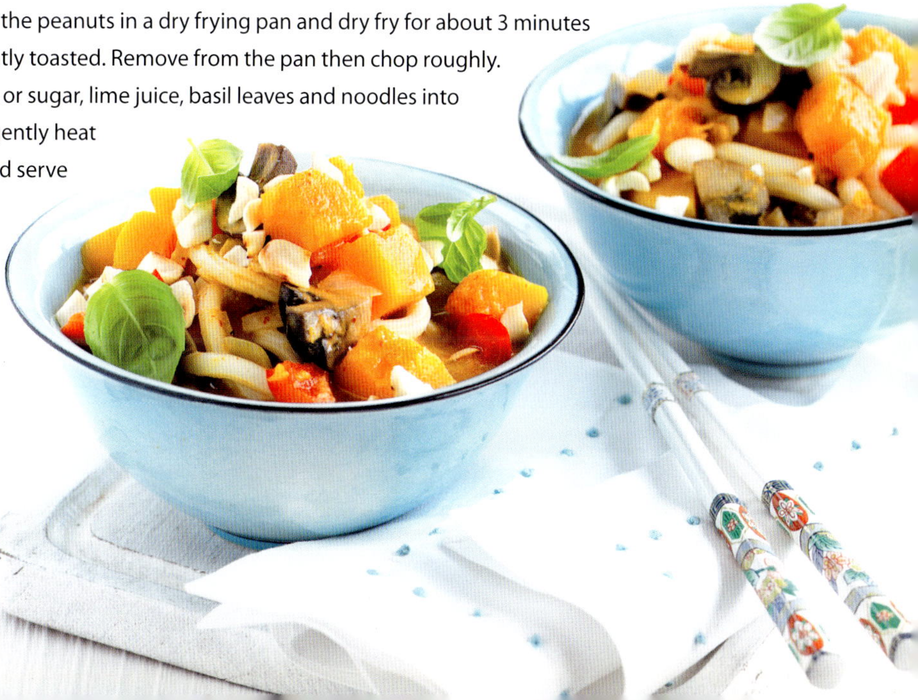

ProPoints values per recipe....... 6
Takes 25 mins

Serves 1

50 g (1¾ oz) dried vermicelli rice noodles
½ a kettleful of boiling water
50 g (1¾ oz) **broccoli** florets
4 **baby corn**
3 **asparagus** tips
1 small **carrot**, peeled and sliced thinly into rounds
2 chestnut **mushrooms**, sliced thinly
250 ml (9 fl oz) vegetable stock
½ teaspoon lemongrass paste
½ teaspoon finely chopped **fresh root ginger**
1 **spring onion**, sliced diagonally
1 tablespoon fish sauce
1 tablespoon light soy sauce
½ teaspoon fructose or caster sugar
a large pinch of dried chilli flakes

To garnish
2 **watercress** sprigs, trimmed
a few **coriander leaves**

Vegetable noodle soup

6 *ProPoints* value

This typically Thai soup is deliciously satisfying with plenty of vegetables and noodles.

1 Put the noodles in a bowl and pour over enough boiling water to just cover them. Stir, then leave for 10 minutes until tender. Drain the noodles then return them to the bowl and cover with cold water. Set aside.

2 Meanwhile, bring about 2.5 cm (1 inch) of water to the boil in a lidded pan. Put the broccoli, baby corn, asparagus and carrot in a steamer basket and place it over the pan. Cover and steam for 3 minutes until nearly tender. Alternatively, bring a small amount of water to the boil and cook the vegetables for 3 minutes then drain. Refresh the vegetables under cold running water and set aside.

3 Put the mushrooms, stock, lemongrass paste, ginger, spring onion, fish sauce, soy sauce, fructose or sugar and chilli flakes in a saucepan, stir and bring to the boil. Reduce the heat and add the vegetables and drained noodles, then heat through briefly.

4 Pour into a serving bowl and garnish with the watercress and coriander.

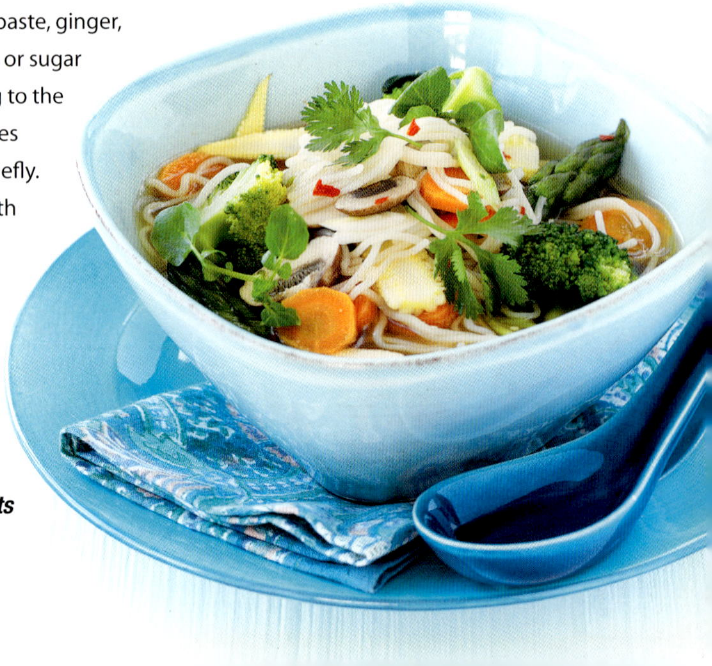

V Cook's tip It's possible to buy vegetarian fish sauce, if preferred, from oriental shops or online.

Variation Add 125 g (4½ oz) cooked **skinless boneless chicken breast**, cut into strips in step 3, for a total of 11 ***ProPoints*** values per serving.

in a wok

With a wok, you can create an amazing variety of meals in minutes. Stir up some tasty Spicy Beef or for something fun and fabulous, try the Vietnamese Coconut Pancakes or the Chinese Egg Rolls.

Teriyaki chicken on page 31

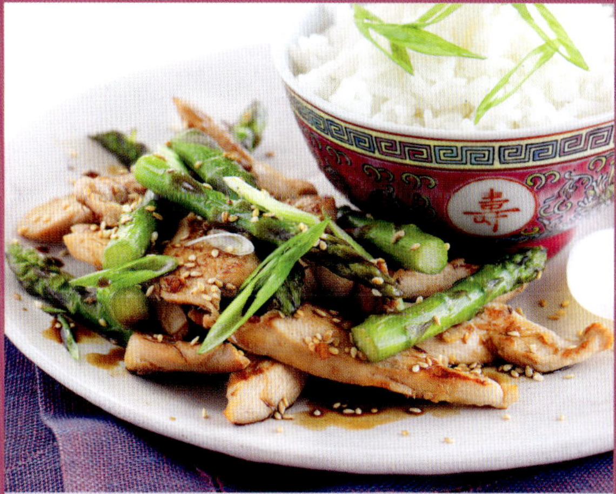

ProPoints **values per serving** 6
ProPoints **values per recipe** 25
Takes 20 mins

Serves 4

2 tablespoons soy sauce
2 tablespoons smooth peanut butter
low fat cooking spray
2 large **garlic cloves**, chopped
2.5 cm (1 inch) **fresh root ginger**, chopped finely
125 g (4½ oz) **mange tout**
350 g (12 oz) **Quorn pieces**
1 teaspoon ground turmeric
100 ml (3½ fl oz) vegetable stock
200 ml (7 fl oz) light coconut milk
1 red **chilli**, de-seeded and sliced thinly into rounds (optional)
2 tablespoons lime juice
60 g (2 oz) **beansprouts**
2 **spring onions**, sliced diagonally
salt and freshly ground black pepper

Malay style Quorn

6 *ProPoints* value

Serve with 60 g (2 oz) dried rice noodles per person, cooked according to the packet instructions, for an additional 6 ***ProPoints*** values per serving.

1. Mix together the soy sauce, peanut butter and 3 tablespoons of hot water in a small bowl. Set aside.
2. Heat a wok or non stick frying pan until hot. Spray with the cooking spray and stir fry the garlic, ginger and mange tout for 1 minute then add the Quorn pieces and turmeric.
3. Pour in the stock, coconut milk and chilli, if using, and bring to the boil then reduce the heat and simmer for 5 minutes. Stir in the soy sauce mixture and lime juice, season to taste, then add the beansprouts just before serving.
4. Serve in warm shallow bowls, sprinkled with the spring onions.

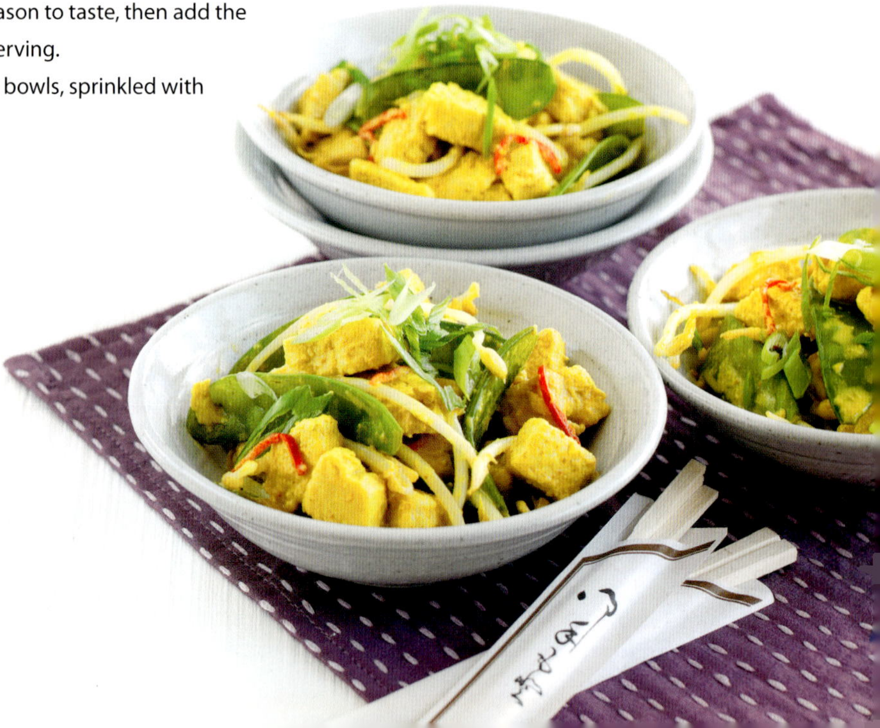

ProPoints **values per serving 4**
ProPoints **values per recipe 17**
Takes 25 mins

Serves 4

400 g (14 oz) pork tenderloin, visible fat removed, and cut into strips
4 tablespoons dark soy sauce
low fat cooking spray
1 onion, sliced thinly
75 g (2¾ oz) baby corn, halved lengthways
1 yellow pepper, de-seeded and cut into thin strips
100 g (3½ oz) mange tout, halved diagonally
1 red chilli, de-seeded and cut into rounds
1 teaspoon ground turmeric
1 tablespoon brown sugar
juice of 1 lime
½ teaspoon cornflour, mixed with a little water
50 g (1¾ oz) beansprouts

Singapore pork

This simple weekday meal can be rustled up in a matter of minutes.

1 Put the pork and soy sauce in a shallow dish and turn until the meat is coated. Set aside.

2 Heat a wok or large non stick frying pan until hot. Spray with the cooking spray and stir fry the onion and baby corn for 3 minutes. Add the yellow pepper and mange tout and stir fry for another minute. Transfer to a bowl while you cook the pork.

3 Remove the pork from the soy sauce, add to the pan, spray with the cooking spray, and stir fry for 3 minutes. Mix the chilli, turmeric, sugar, lime juice and cornflour mixture into the soy sauce, add to the pan, spray with cooking spray and then stir fry for 1 minute.

4 Return the cooked vegetables to the pan and add the beansprouts. Stir briefly until combined, then serve.

V Variation You can use 350 g (12 oz) **Quorn pieces** instead of the pork in this recipe for 3 ***ProPoints*** values per serving. Prepare and cook in the same way as the pork.

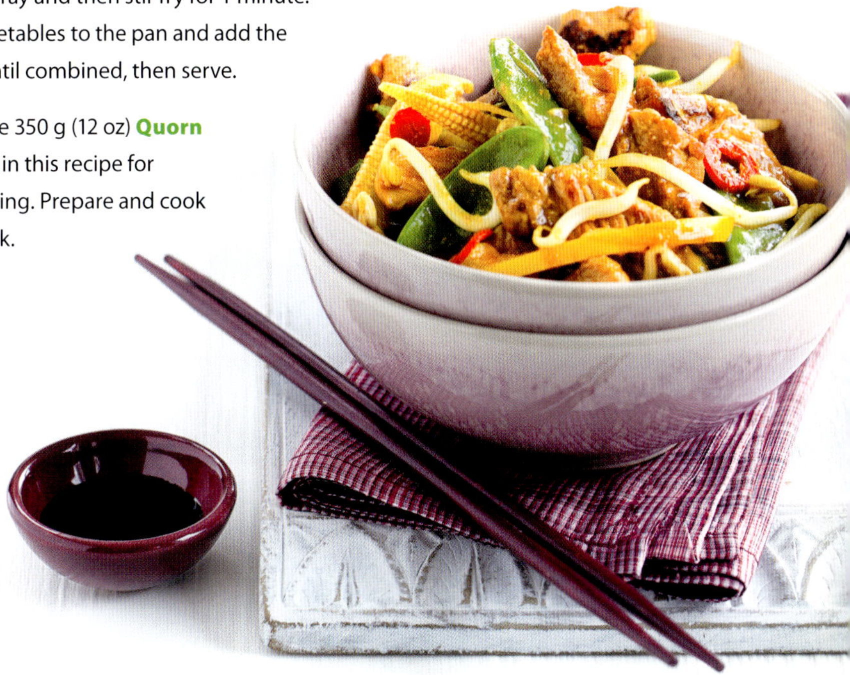

ProPoints values per serving **5**
ProPoints values per recipe **11**
Takes 15 mins

Serves 2

2 tablespoons soy sauce
2 tablespoons orange juice
½ teaspoon sugar
1 teaspoon cornflour
½ teaspoon Szechuan pepper
250 g (9 oz) lean beef strips
low fat cooking spray
½ red pepper, de-seeded and sliced
2 pak choi, sliced roughly crossways
2 large garlic cloves, chopped

Spicy beef

5 *ProPoints* value

Szechuan pepper adds a distinctively warm and slight lemony flavour to this beef stir fry. Serve with 50 g (1¾ oz) dried egg noodles per person, cooked according to the packet instructions, for an additional 6 ***ProPoints*** values per serving.

1. Mix together the soy sauce, orange juice and sugar. In a separate bowl, stir the cornflour into 2 tablespoons of cold water. Set both mixtures aside to use later.
2. Put the Szechuan pepper in a dry wok or non stick frying pan and dry fry for about 1 minute then remove and grind with a pestle and mortar until it is a coarse powder.
3. Spray the beef with the cooking spray, add to the pan and then stir fry for 2 minutes. Remove from the pan and set aside. Add the red pepper, the white part of the pak choi and the garlic to the pan and then stir fry for 1 minute.
4. Stir the cornflour mixture again. Return the beef to the pan with the green part of the pak choi, the ground Szechuan pepper, the soy sauce mixture and the cornflour. Stir fry for a minute until heated through and the sauce is thickened and glossy. Serve immediately.

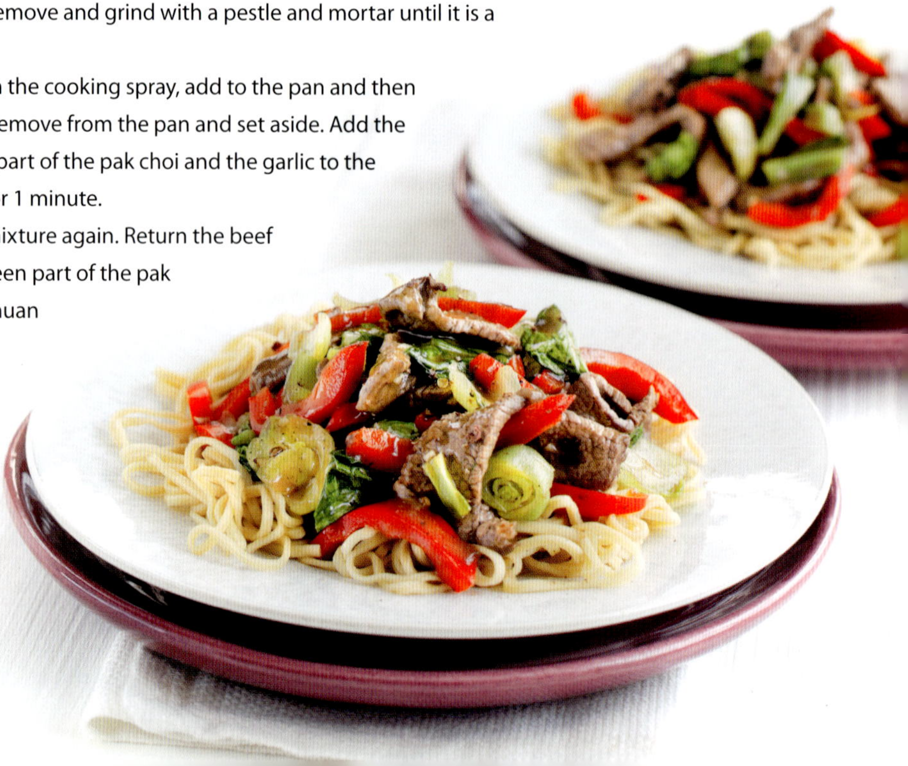

ProPoints **values per serving 10**
ProPoints **values per recipe 21**
Takes 20 mins + 15 mins marinating
Serves 2

3 tablespoons hoisin sauce
2 tablespoons dark soy sauce
200 g (7 oz) skinless boneless duck breasts, visible fat removed then cut into strips
125 g (4½ oz) small **broccoli** florets
100 g (3½ oz) frozen **soya beans**
low fat cooking spray
1 **spring onion**, sliced diagonally
freshly ground black pepper

Hoisin duck stir fry

Serve with three warmed Chinese pancakes per person for an additional 3 ***ProPoints*** values per serving. You'll find them in the freezer cabinet in supermarkets, or in oriental shops.

1 Mix together the hoisin and soy sauces in a shallow dish. Add the duck and turn until coated then set aside for 15 minutes.

2 Meanwhile, bring a pan of water to the boil and blanch the broccoli for 2 minutes then add the soya beans and cook for another 1 minute. Drain and refresh under cold running water. Set aside.

3 Heat a wok or non stick frying pan until hot. Remove the duck from the marinade, add to the wok or pan and spray with the cooking spray. Stir fry for 3 minutes then add the broccoli, soya beans, hoisin sauce mixture and 2 tablespoons of water. Stir fry for another minute, season with black pepper and serve in bowls with the spring onion scattered over the top.

Variation You can swap the duck for 200 g (7 oz) **tofu**, patted dry and cut into squares for 10 ***ProPoints*** values per serving. Marinate and cook in the same way as the duck.

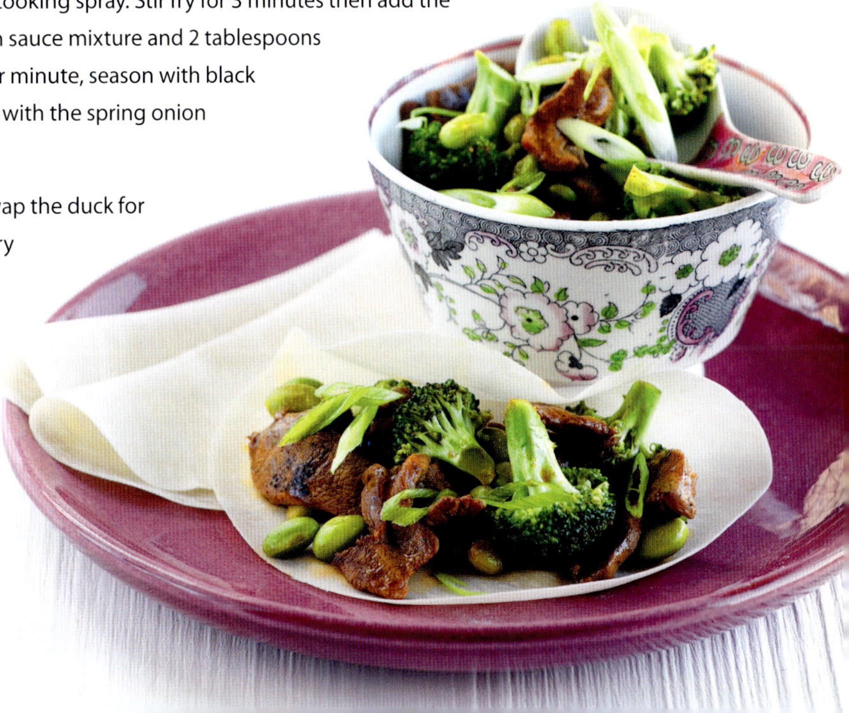

ProPoints values per serving 7
ProPoints values per recipe 27
Takes 30 mins

Serves 4

- 3 tablespoons light soy sauce
- 4 teaspoons clear honey
- grated zest and juice of 1 small lemon
- 2 teaspoons cornflour
- 40 g (1½ oz) cashew nuts
- low fat cooking spray
- 500 g (1 lb 2 oz) **skinless boneless chicken breast**, cut into strips
- 1 **onion**, sliced
- 2.5 cm (1 inch) **fresh root ginger**, chopped finely
- 100 g (3½ oz) **baby corn**, halved lengthways
- 125 g (4½ oz) **sugar snap peas**

Lemon & ginger chicken

7 *ProPoints* value

This delicious dish features the lovely combination of fresh lemon juice, ginger and honey.

1 Mix together the soy sauce, honey, lemon zest and juice, and cornflour in a shallow dish.

2 Put the cashews in a dry wok or non stick frying pan and dry fry, turning occasionally, for 3–4 minutes until light golden. Set aside.

3 Heat a wok or non stick frying pan until hot, spray the chicken with the cooking spray and stir fry for 5–6 minutes until golden all over. Remove from the pan and transfer the chicken to the soy sauce mixture and turn until coated.

4 Spray the pan with the cooking spray and stir fry the onion for 3 minutes. Add the ginger, baby corn and sugar snap peas then cook for another 2 minutes.

5 Return the chicken to the pan with the soy mixture and stir fry for 1–2 minutes until the sauce is reduced and thickened. Serve topped with the toasted cashews.

V Variation You can replace the chicken with 350 g (12 oz) **Quorn pieces**. Marinate in the soy mixture for 15 minutes then add to the stir fry in step 4 with the onion. The *ProPoints* values per serving will be 6.

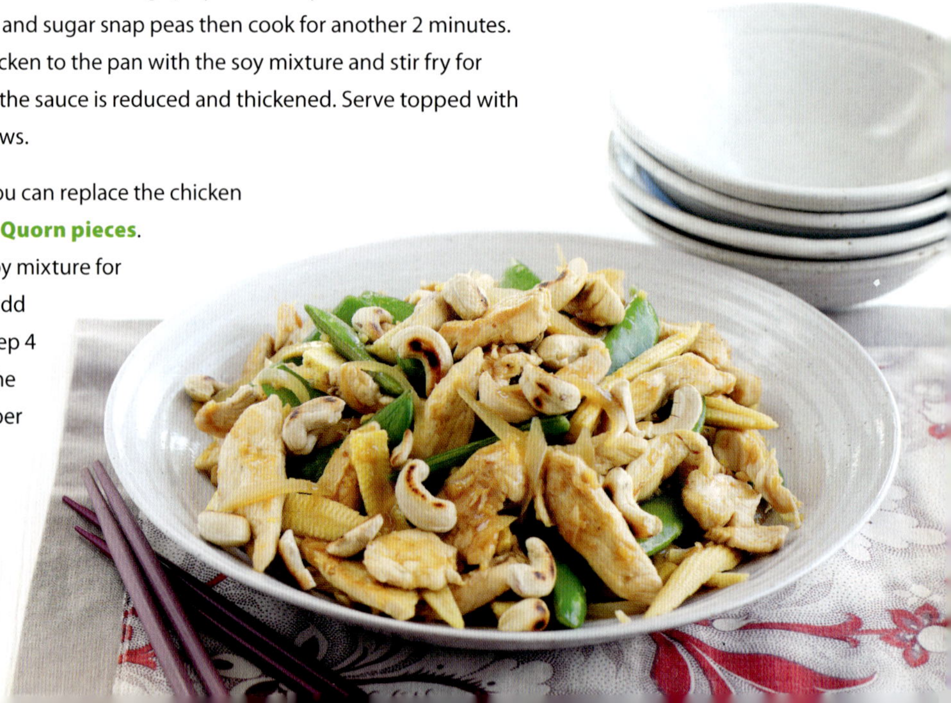

***ProPoints* values per serving** 5
***ProPoints* values per recipe** 18
Takes 20 mins + 30 mins marinating

Serves 4

- 4 tablespoons teriyaki marinade
- 1 tablespoon light soy sauce
- ½ teaspoon toasted sesame oil
- 500 g (1 lb 2 oz) **skinless boneless chicken breast**, cut into strips
- 2 teaspoons sesame seeds
- low fat cooking spray
- 250 g (9 oz) **asparagus tips**
- 2.5 cm (1 inch) **fresh root ginger**, chopped finely
- 2 **spring onions**, sliced diagonally

Teriyaki chicken

Serve with 60 g (2 oz) dried jasmine rice per person, cooked according to the packet instructions, for an additional 6 ***ProPoints*** values per serving.

1. Mix together the teriyaki marinade, soy sauce and sesame oil in a shallow dish. Add the chicken, stir until coated, and leave to marinate for 30 minutes.
2. Meanwhile, put the sesame seeds in a dry wok or non stick frying pan and dry fry for about 3 minutes, shaking the pan occasionally, until light golden. Set aside.
3. Remove the chicken from the marinade (reserving the marinade for later), spray with the cooking spray, add to the pan and stir fry for 5–6 minutes until light golden all over. Remove from the pan and set aside.
4. Spray the pan with the cooking spray and stir fry the asparagus for 3 minutes then add the ginger, chicken and the reserved marinade. Stir fry for a further 1–2 minutes until the sauce is reduced and thickened. Serve sprinkled with the sesame seeds and spring onions.

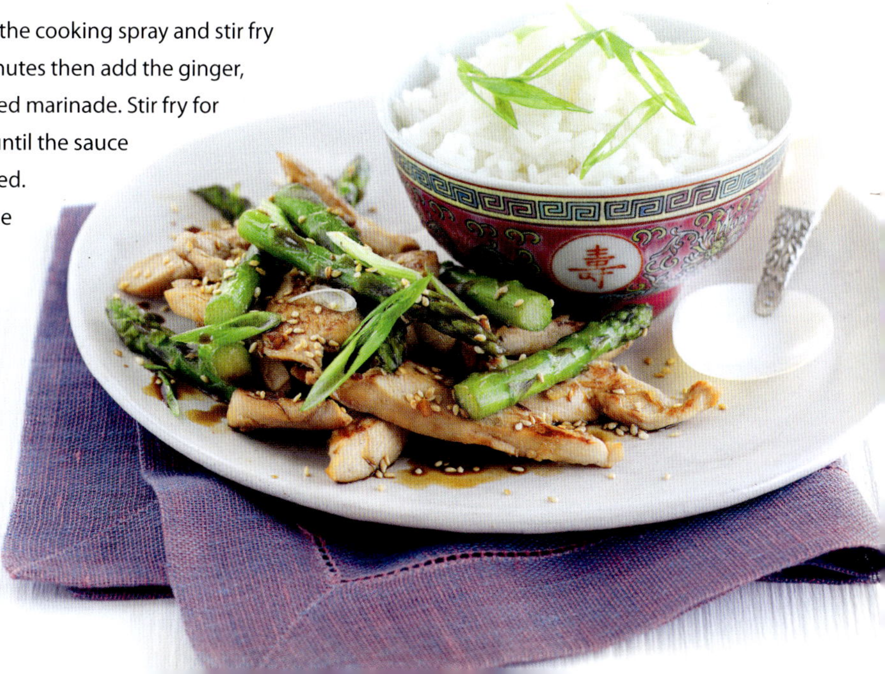

Chinese egg rolls with prawns

5 *ProPoints* value

***ProPoints* values per recipe** 5
Takes 25 mins

Serves 1

- 40 g (1½ oz) tenderstem **broccoli**, trimmed
- low fat cooking spray
- 40 g (1½ oz) **Chinese leaves**, shredded
- ¼ small red **pepper**, de-seeded and sliced into strips
- 1 large **spring onion**, cut into strips
- 1 **garlic clove**, chopped
- 1 teaspoon chopped **fresh root ginger**
- 50 g (1¾ oz) small cooked **prawns**
- 1 tablespoon black bean sauce
- 1 teaspoon light soy sauce
- 1 large **egg**, lightly beaten
- salt and freshly ground black pepper

Serve with 50 g (1¾ oz) dried egg noodles, cooked according to the packet instructions, for an additional 6 ***ProPoints*** values.

1. Bring about 2.5 cm (1 inch) of water to the boil in a lidded pan. Put the broccoli in a steamer basket and place it over the pan. Cover and steam for 2 minutes until almost tender. Alternatively, bring a small amount of water to the boil and cook the broccoli for 2 minutes then drain. Refresh the broccoli under cold running water and set aside.
2. Meanwhile, heat a lidded wok or non stick frying pan until hot. Spray with the cooking spray then stir fry the Chinese leaves, red pepper, spring onion, garlic and ginger for 2 minutes.
3. Add the broccoli, prawns, black bean sauce and soy sauce then heat through for 1 minute, stirring. Cover to keep warm while you make the omelette.
4. Heat a medium size, non stick frying pan. Spray with the cooking spray, season the egg and then pour into the pan. Swirl the pan until the egg coats the bottom in an even layer. Cook for about 2 minutes until set, then slide the omelette on to a plate, using a spatula to help.
5. Spoon the vegetable and prawn mixture down the centre of the omelette then roll up. Cut in half on the diagonal to serve.

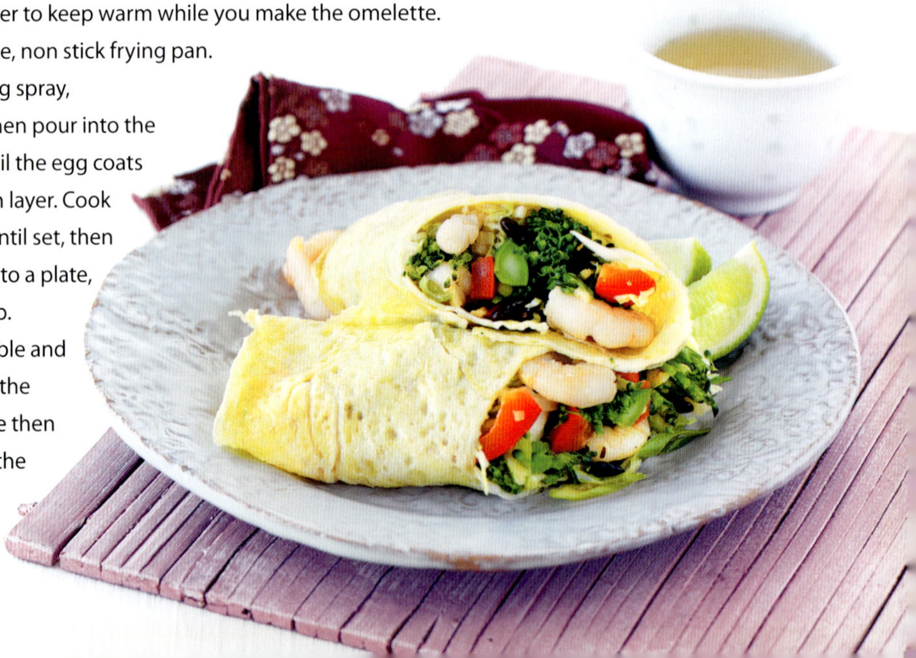

Beef & broccoli stir fry

6 *ProPoints* value

***ProPoints* values per recipe** 6
Takes 20 mins

Serves 1

2 tablespoons oyster sauce
1 tablespoon dark soy sauce
125 g (4½ oz) **lean beef fillet**, cut into thin strips
low fat cooking spray
80 g (3 oz) tenderstem **broccoli**, trimmed
1 **carrot**, peeled and cut into batons
2 **spring onions**, sliced diagonally
2 **garlic cloves**, chopped
15 g (½ oz) **fresh root ginger**, cut into matchsticks
½ red **chilli**, de-seeded and chopped

Serve with 150 g (5½ oz) straight-to-wok rice noodles for an additional 5 ***ProPoints*** values per serving, for an easy meal for one.

1 Mix together the oyster sauce and soy sauce in a dish and add the beef, turning until coated. Set aside.

2 Heat a wok or non stick frying pan until hot. Spray with the cooking spray and stir fry the broccoli and carrot for 3 minutes. Add the white part of the spring onions (reserving the green part), garlic and ginger and stir fry for 30 seconds. Remove from the pan and set aside.

3 Remove the beef from the marinade, add to the pan and spray with the cooking spray. Stir fry for 2 minutes before returning the vegetables to the pan with the marinade, chilli and 1 tablespoon of water. Heat through and scatter over the green part of the spring onion before serving.

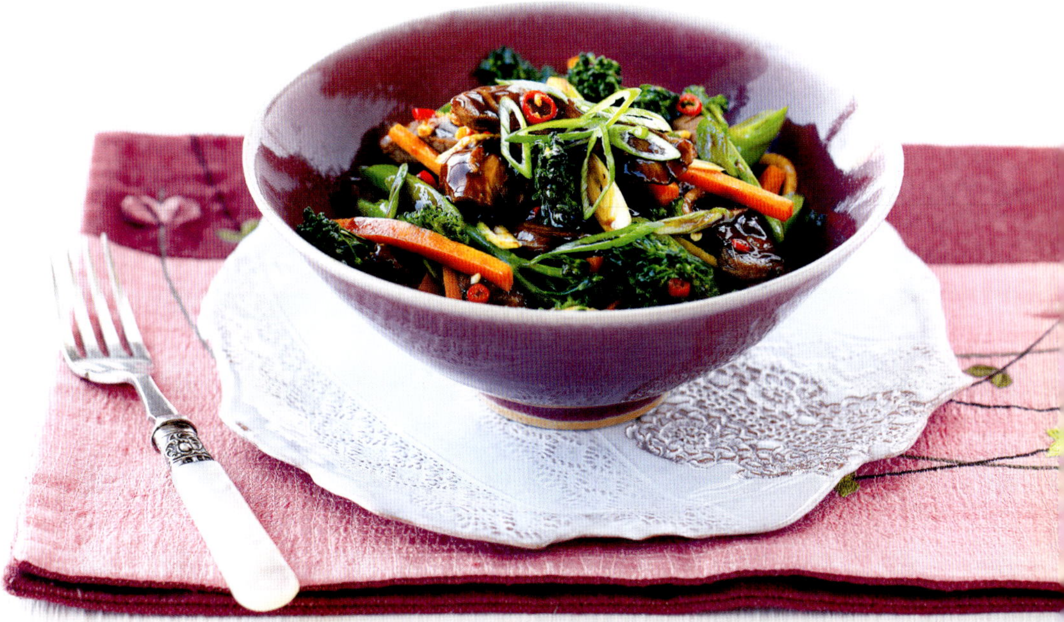

Vietnamese coconut pancakes with veggies

4 *ProPoints* value

ProPoints **values per serving 4**
ProPoints **values per recipe 14**
Takes 45 mins + 30 mins resting

pancakes only — **Serves 4**

1 tablespoon light soy sauce
1 tablespoon fish sauce
1 tablespoon lime juice
1 teaspoon caster sugar
low fat cooking spray
1 onion, sliced
1 large carrot, peeled and sliced diagonally
1 large courgette, sliced diagonally
2 pak choi, sliced
100 g (3½ oz) portobello mushrooms, sliced
1 large garlic clove, chopped
a large pinch of dried chilli flakes

For the coconut pancakes

90 g (3¼ oz) plain flour
½ teaspoon baking powder
½ teaspoon ground turmeric
a large pinch of salt
100 ml (3½ fl oz) light coconut milk
1 egg

This delicious recipe is easy and makes a nice change for a simple supper.

1 To make the pancakes, sift the flour, baking powder, turmeric and salt into a mixing bowl. Mix the coconut milk with 150 ml (5 fl oz) water in a jug then beat in the egg. Gradually whisk the liquid mixture into the dry ingredients to make a smooth batter. Set aside in the fridge for 30 minutes.

2 Mix together the soy sauce, fish sauce, lime juice, sugar and 1 tablespoon of water.

3 Heat a large non stick frying pan and spray with the cooking spray. Pour 40 ml (1½ fl oz) of the batter into the pan. Tip the pan until the batter covers the bottom in a thin layer then cook for about 1½–2 minutes on each side until light golden. Keep warm while you make the remaining seven pancakes.

4 Heat a wok or non stick frying pan until hot then spray with the cooking spray. Stir fry the onion for 1 minute then add the carrot, courgette, pak choi, mushrooms, garlic and chilli flakes for another 2–3 minutes.

5 Pour in the soy mixture and stir fry for 1–2 minutes until the liquid is reduced. Serve two pancakes per person and top with the vegetables.

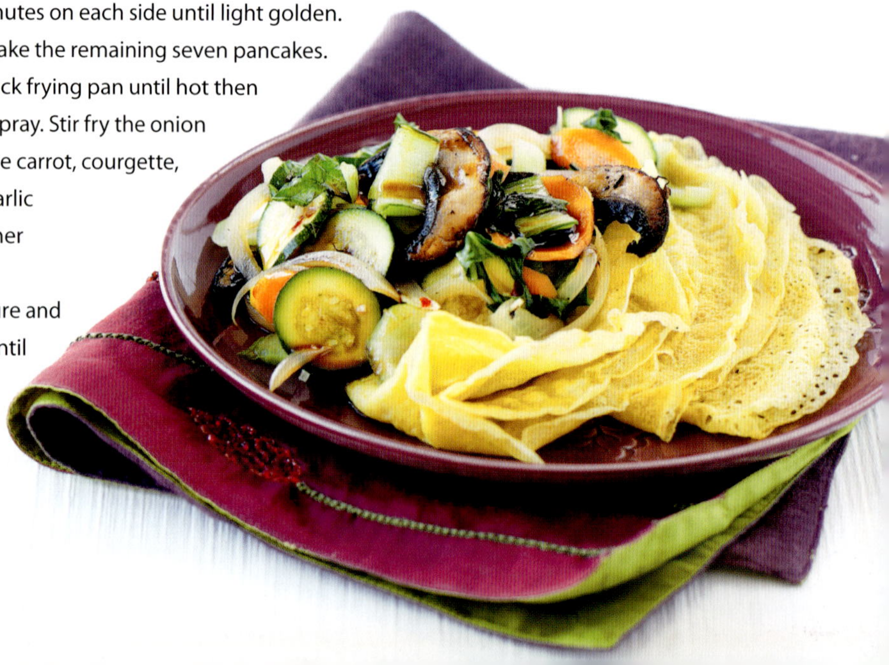

grills and roasts

You'll love making these tasty grills and roasts. They're so easy and with such exotic and satisfying flavours, they're sure to be a hit with everyone.

Szechuan orange pork on page 42

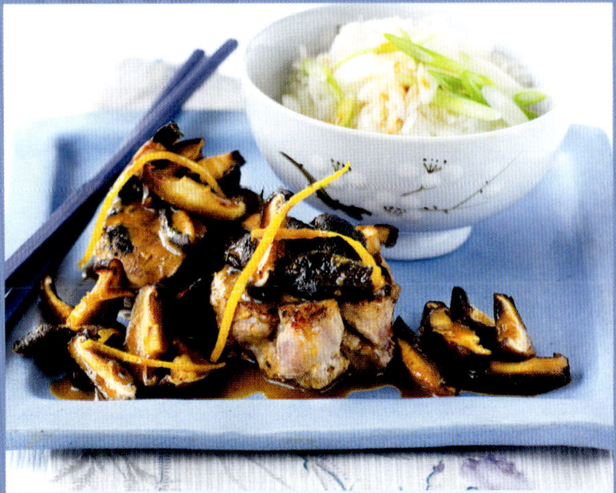

Aromatic lamb with mint relish

8 *ProPoints* value

ProPoints **values per serving 8**
ProPoints **values per recipe 33**
20 mins prep + 1 hr marinating, 50 mins cooking

Serves 4

600 g (1 lb 5 oz) boneless leg of lamb, visible fat removed
4 cm (1½ inches) fresh root ginger
2 tablespoons plum sauce
2 tablespoons dark soy sauce
2 large garlic cloves, sliced thinly
salt and freshly ground black pepper

For the fresh mint relish

3 tablespoons extra light mayonnaise
1 tablespoon rice vinegar
15 g (½ oz) fresh mint leaves, chopped roughly
2 teaspoons mint sauce

Serve with plenty of zero ***ProPoints*** value vegetables, such as **carrots** and **runner beans**. For roasted potatoes, roast 400 g (14 oz) **new potatoes** in 2 tablespoons of olive oil and serve 100 g (3½ oz) per person, for an additional 4 ***ProPoints*** values per serving.

1 Heat the oven to Gas Mark 6/200°C/fan oven 180°C. Make cuts diagonally across the lamb. Grate one half of the ginger and, using your hands, squeeze out the juice into a bowl. Discard the remaining fibrous bits of ginger. Mix in the plum sauce and soy sauce. Put the lamb in a dish and spoon over the marinade making sure the meat is well covered.

2 Thinly slice the remaining ginger and press well into the cuts in the lamb. Repeat with the garlic. Season well and set aside for at least 1 hour to marinate.

3 Put the lamb in a roasting tin and spoon over any excess marinade. Roast for 50 minutes, spooning over any marinade halfway through, until the top is dark golden and glossy.

4 Meanwhile, make the relish. Mix together the mayonnaise, rice vinegar, fresh mint and mint sauce. Season then set aside until ready to use. When the lamb is cooked, let it rest for 10 minutes then carve into slices and serve with the mint relish.

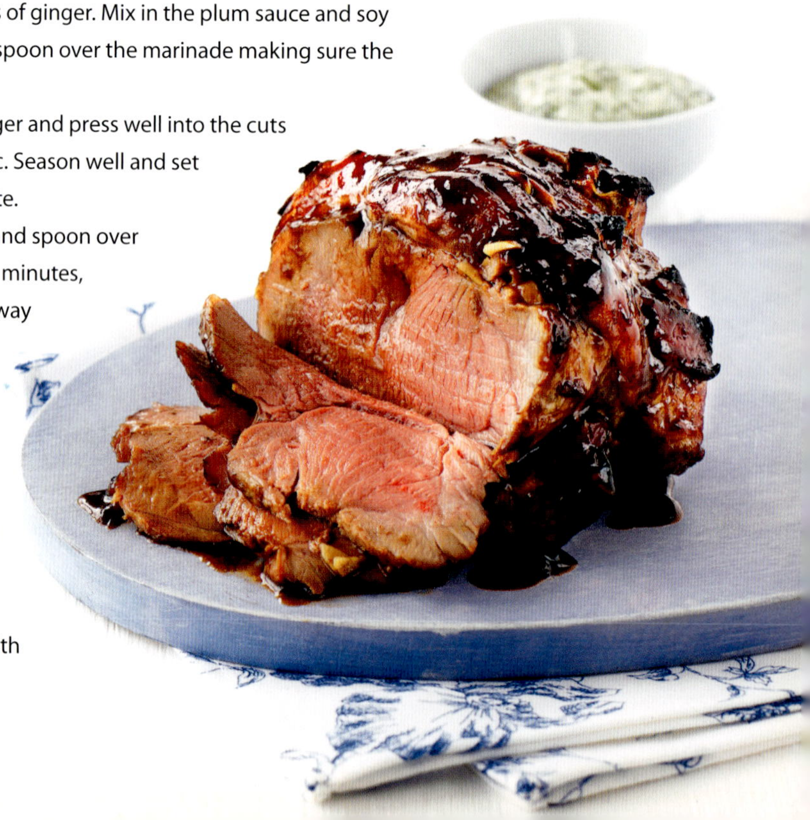

ProPoints **values per serving 5**
ProPoints **values per recipe 21**
Takes 20 mins + 1 hr marinating

Serves 4

400 g (14 oz) **lean beef fillet**, visible fat removed
2 tablespoons plum sauce
2 tablespoons dark soy sauce
2 tablespoons sweet chilli sauce
salt and freshly ground black pepper
4 lime wedges, to garnish

For the oriental slaw

2 teaspoons sesame seeds
100 g (3½ oz) red **cabbage**, shredded
2 **carrots**, peeled and grated
3 **spring onions**, sliced thinly
1 teaspoon toasted sesame oil
1 tablespoon rice vinegar

Plum & sweet chilli beef kebabs

5 *ProPoints* value

For a wonderful smoky flavour, you could also cook these beef kebabs on the barbecue.

1 If using wooden skewers, soak four in water for 30 minutes first to prevent them from burning. Flatten the beef with the end of a rolling pin then cut into 12 x 2 cm (¾ inch) wide strips. Mix together the plum sauce, soy sauce and sweet chilli sauce in a shallow dish and season well. Add the beef and stir until the meat is coated in the marinade. Cover and leave to marinate for 1 hour.

2 Meanwhile, make the oriental slaw. Dry fry the sesame seeds in a dry frying pan for 3 minutes until light golden. Put the cabbage, carrots and spring onions in a serving bowl. Mix together the sesame oil and rice vinegar, season, then pour it over the slaw. Turn until coated in the dressing then sprinkle over the sesame seeds.

3 Preheat the grill to high. Thread the beef on to the four skewers and spoon over some of the marinade. Grill for 2 minutes then turn the kebabs, spoon over more of the marinade and cook for another 2 minutes. Serve the kebabs with the oriental slaw, garnished with lime wedges for squeezing over.

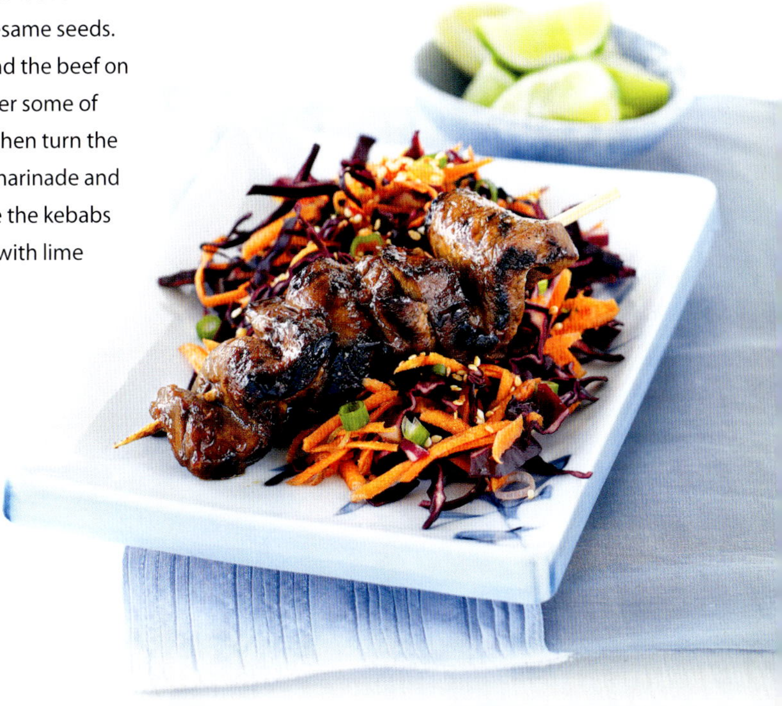

Indian stuffed peppers

ProPoints values per serving 4
ProPoints values per recipe 18
30 mins prep, 40 mins cooking

Serves 4

400 g (14 oz) **potatoes**, peeled and halved or quartered, if large
4 red **peppers**
low fat cooking spray
1 large **onion**, diced
2 **courgettes**, diced
3 large **garlic cloves**, chopped
2 tablespoons balti spice paste

For the ginger tomato sauce

300 ml (10 fl oz) **passata**
½ teaspoon sugar
2.5 cm (1 inch) **fresh root ginger**, grated
salt and freshly ground black pepper

1 Bring a large pan of water to the boil and cook the potatoes for about 10 minutes or until tender. Drain, set aside to cool slightly, then dice.

2 Meanwhile, put the peppers in a large saucepan of water and bring to the boil, then reduce the heat and simmer for 4 minutes until softened. Using a slotted spoon, carefully remove the peppers from the water and set aside until cool enough to handle. Slice the top off each pepper to make a lid, scoop out the seeds then turn upside down to drain.

3 Preheat the oven to Gas Mark 5/190°C/fan oven 170°C. Heat a wok or non stick frying pan until hot. Spray with the cooking spray and stir fry the onion, courgettes and garlic for 3 minutes. Remove from the heat then stir in the balti spice paste, 4 tablespoons of water and the potatoes. Spoon the mixture into the peppers and top with their lids.

4 Arrange the peppers close together in an ovenproof dish, spray with cooking spray and pour 3 tablespoons of water into the dish. Cover with foil and bake in the oven for 40 minutes.

5 To make the ginger tomato sauce, spray a saucepan with the cooking spray, add the passata and sugar and bring to the boil. Reduce the heat and simmer for 10 minutes until reduced and thickened. Squeeze the juice from the ginger into the pan. Discard the fibrous bits of ginger. Season, stir and heat through. Serve with the sauce on the side.

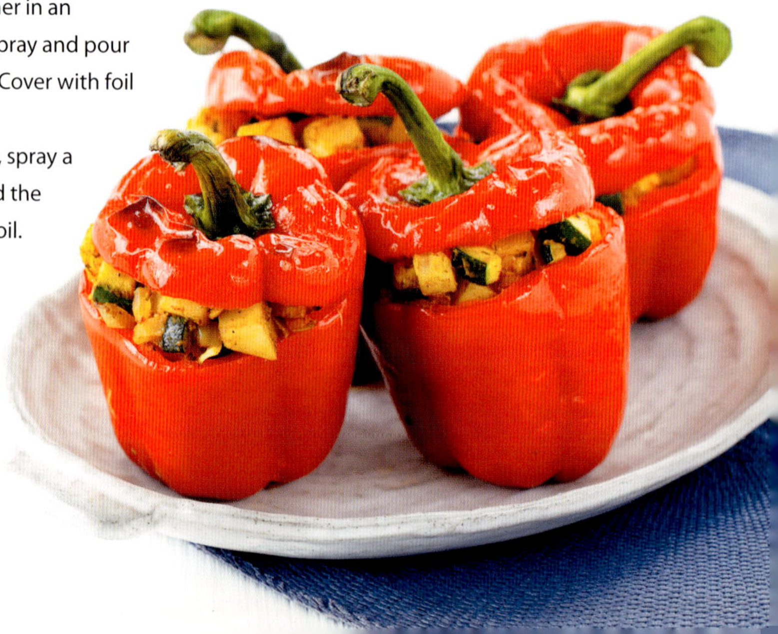

ProPoints values per serving 6
ProPoints values per recipe 11
Takes 25 mins

Serves 2

½ teaspoon toasted sesame oil
2 tablespoons teriyaki marinade
1 tablespoon light soy sauce
2 x 150 g (5½ oz) skinless boneless chicken breasts
1 cm (½ inch) fresh root ginger, sliced into rounds
2 spring onions, shredded
½ teaspoon sesame seeds
2 carrots, peeled and cut into ribbons using a vegetable peeler
2 teaspoons lime juice

For the wasabi dip

4 teaspoons extra light mayonnaise
2 teaspoons wasabi paste

Sesame chicken parcels

6 ProPoints value

Cooking the chicken in a parcel helps to keep it moist and succulent; it's also one of the easiest ways to cook fish.

1 Preheat the oven to Gas Mark 6/200°C/fan oven 180°C. Mix together the sesame oil, teriyaki marinade and soy sauce.

2 Place each chicken breast on a piece of foil, large enough to make a parcel. Spoon over the teriyaki mixture then arrange the ginger and spring onions on top. Fold over the foil and seal to make two loose parcels then place on a baking sheet.

3 Bake in the oven for 20 minutes until the chicken is cooked through and there is no trace of pink in the centre. While the chicken is cooking, dry fry the sesame seeds by putting them in a dry non stick frying pan and dry frying them over a medium heat, shaking the pan occasionally, for about 3 minutes until light golden.

4 Mix together both of the ingredients for the wasabi dip with 1 teaspoon of warm water.

5 Carefully open each parcel on to a plate. Arrange the carrots by the side, squeeze over the lime juice and sprinkle with the sesame seeds. Serve with a spoonful of the wasabi dip.

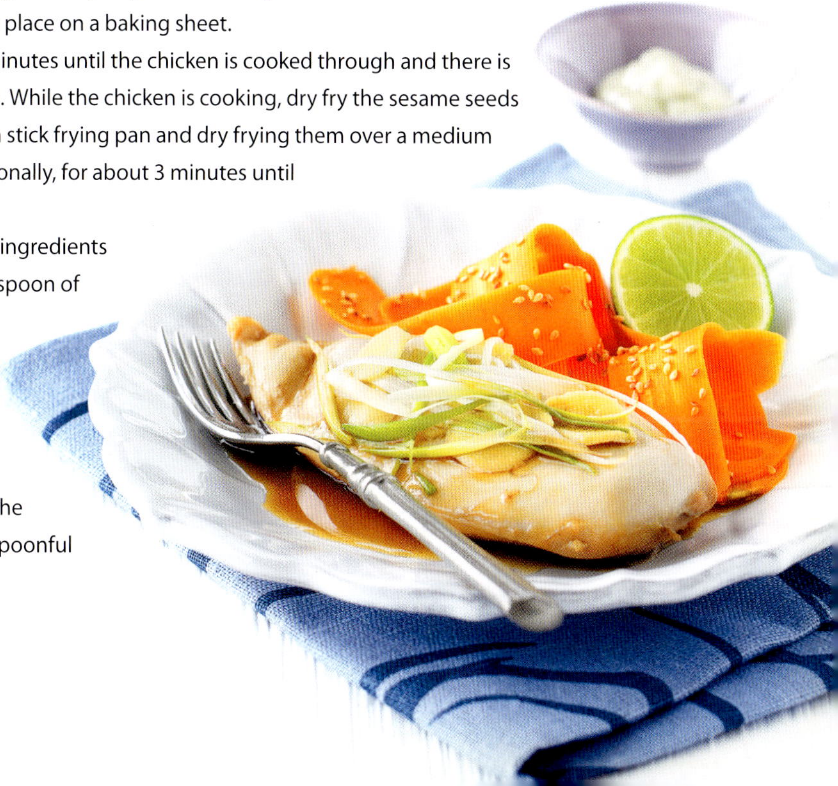

***ProPoints* values per serving** 5
***ProPoints* values per recipe** 11
20 mins prep + 30 mins chilling,
12 mins cooking

Serves 2

- 250 g (9 oz) lean turkey mince
- 2 teaspoons grated **fresh root ginger**
- 2 kaffir lime leaves, shredded finely
- 1 teaspoon lemongrass paste
- 3 **spring onions**, chopped
- 3 tablespoons **fresh coriander**, chopped finely
- 1 red **chilli**, de-seeded and chopped finely
- 1 **egg white**
- low fat cooking spray
- salt and freshly ground black pepper

For the pea shoot salad

- 40 g (1½ oz) **pea shoots**
- 25 g (1 oz) baby **spinach leaves**, tough stalks removed
- 5 **radishes**, trimmed and sliced into rounds
- ½ small red **onion**, sliced thinly
- 1 teaspoon sesame oil
- 1 teaspoon grated **fresh root ginger**
- 1 tablespoon rice vinegar

Thai turkey sticks

5 *ProPoints* value

Serve these koftas with a warmed wholemeal chapatti each for an additional 4 ***ProPoints*** values per serving.

1 If using wooden skewers, soak four in water for 30 minutes in advance to prevent them from burning during grilling. Mix together the turkey mince, ginger, lime leaves, lemongrass paste, spring onions, coriander, chilli and egg white in a bowl. Season well.

2 With damp hands, divide the mixture into four and shape into a long sausage around the skewers then chill for 30 minutes.

3 Preheat the grill to high and line the grill pan with foil. Spray the turkey koftas with the cooking spray then grill for 10–12 minutes, turning occasionally, until cooked through and light golden.

4 Meanwhile, make the salad. Put the pea shoots and spinach in a bowl and top with the radishes and onion. Mix together the sesame oil, ginger and rice vinegar. Season and pour the dressing over the salad. Serve the salad with the cooked koftas.

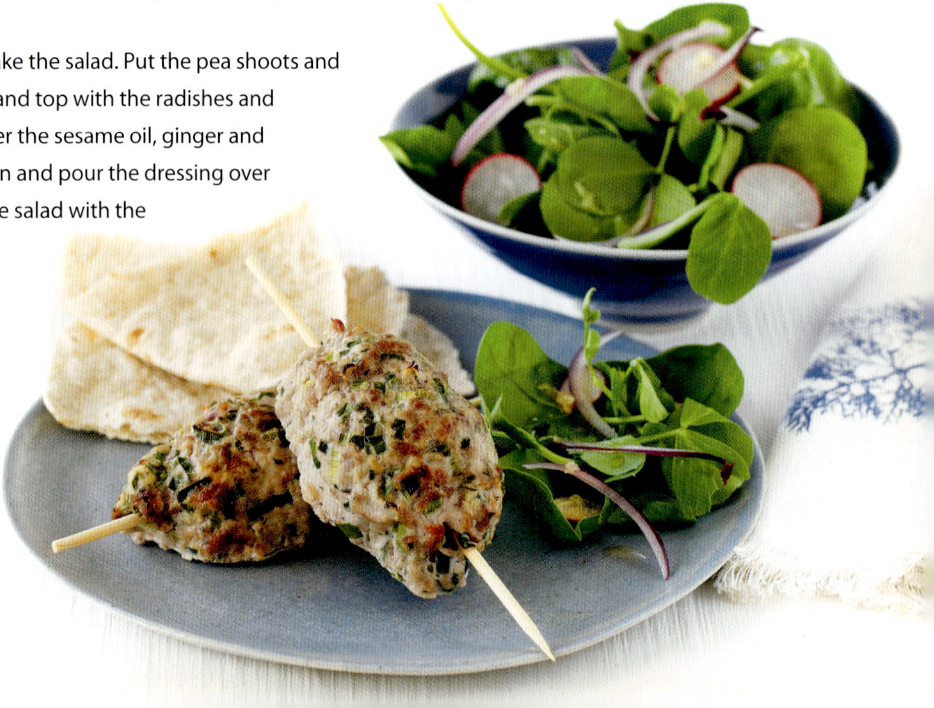

ProPoints values per serving **9**
ProPoints values per recipe **18**
20 mins prep + 30 mins marinating, 10 mins cooking

Serves 2

- 1 tablespoon mirin
- 1 tablespoon light soy sauce
- 1 teaspoon honey
- 2 x 140 g (5 oz) skinless salmon fillets
- 1 Little Gem lettuce, leaves separated
- 40 g (1½ oz) wild rocket leaves
- 5 cm (2 inches) cucumber, halved lengthways and cut into half moons
- ½ small red onion, sliced into rings
- 175 g (6 oz) mango, sliced
- a few fresh mint leaves
- a few fresh basil leaves

For the dressing

- 2 tablespoons fish sauce
- 2 tablespoons lime juice
- 1 tablespoon sweet chilli sauce
- ½ red chilli, de-seeded and chopped
- ½ teaspoon fructose or caster sugar
- salt and freshly ground black pepper

Vietnamese salmon & mango

9 *ProPoints* value

Full of tangy flavours, the salmon in this recipe is complemented by a sweet mango, chilli and hot lime dressing. Serve with 20 g (¾ oz) dried rice noodles per person, cooked according to the packet instructions, for an additional 2 ***ProPoints*** values per serving.

1. Mix together the mirin, soy sauce and honey in a shallow dish. Add the salmon and spoon over the marinade. Set aside for 30 minutes.
2. Meanwhile, make the salad. Arrange the lettuce and rocket leaves on a serving dish and top with the cucumber, red onion and mango.
3. Mix together all the ingredients for the dressing then season.
4. Preheat the grill to high and cover the grill pan with foil. Grill the salmon for 5 minutes on each side until slightly golden, occasionally spooning over the marinade. Leave to cool a little then flake into large pieces.
5. Place the salmon on top of the salad, spoon the dressing over and garnish with the mint and basil leaves. Serve immediately.

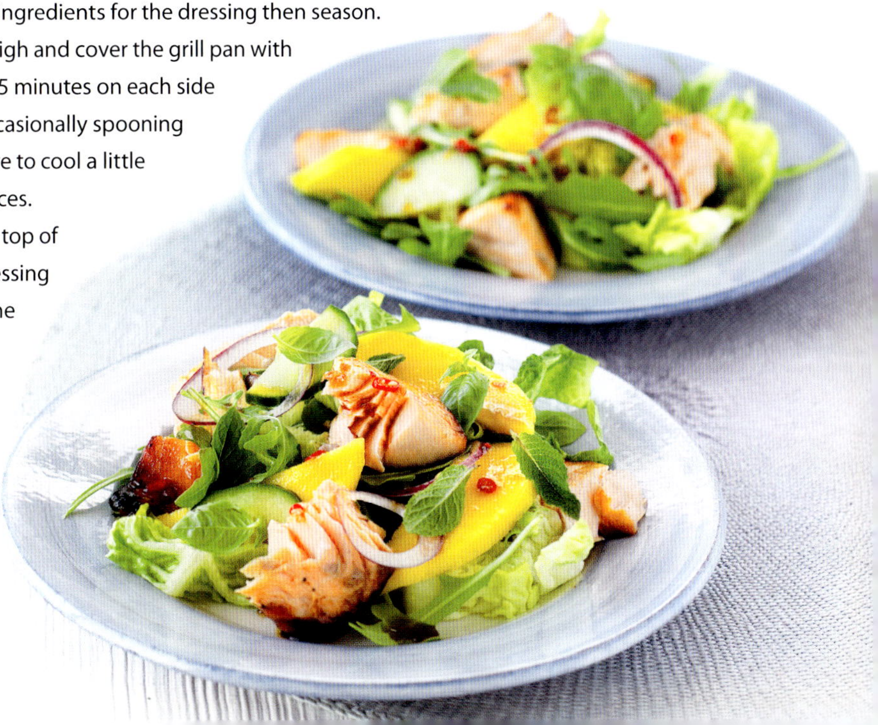

***ProPoints* values per recipe** 9
Takes 25 mins + 30 mins marinating

Serves 1

1 teaspoon clear honey
1 tablespoon light soy sauce
3 tablespoons fresh orange juice
1 tablespoon Chinese cooking wine or dry sherry
140 g (5 oz) **lean pork loin steak**, visible fat removed
low fat cooking spray
60 g (2 oz) shiitake **mushrooms**, stalks removed, sliced
1 cm (½ inch) piece orange zest, cut into very fine strips
salt and freshly ground black pepper
1 **spring onion**, sliced diagonally, to garnish

Szechuan orange pork

9 *ProPoints* value

Serve this aromatic pork and shiitake mushroom dish with 40 g (1½ oz) dried basmati rice, cooked until fluffy, for an additional 4 ***ProPoints*** values.

1 Mix together the honey, soy sauce, orange juice and cooking wine or sherry in a shallow dish. Add the pork, turn to coat it in the marinade, then leave it to marinate for 30 minutes.

2 Preheat the oven to Gas Mark 6/200°C/fan oven 180°C. Heat a non stick frying pan until hot. Remove the pork from the marinade (reserving the marinade for later), put it in the pan and spray with the cooking spray. Brown for 2 minutes on each side. Remove from the pan, loosely wrap in foil and place in a roasting tin. Roast the pork for 10–12 minutes until cooked.

3 Meanwhile, spray the frying pan with the cooking spray. Add the mushrooms then stir fry for 2 minutes. Add the meat marinade, orange zest and any juices from the pork. Bring to the boil and simmer until reduced by half.

4 Season and pour the sauce over the pork. Serve garnished with the spring onion.

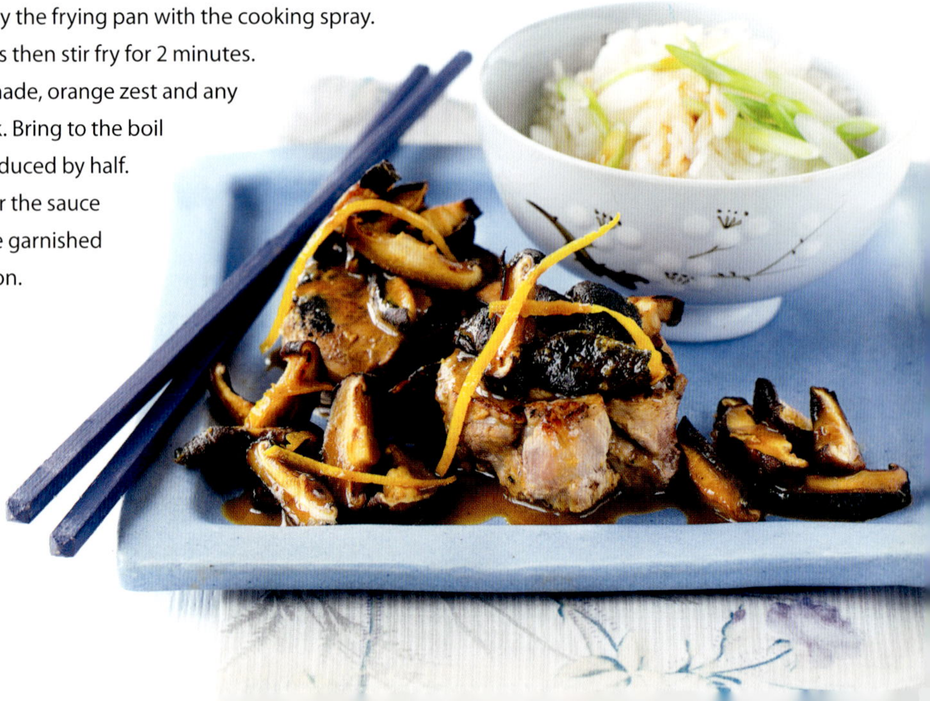

***ProPoints* values per recipe** **4**
Takes 25 mins

Spice crusted fish with vegetable salad

Serves 1

- 1 teaspoon coriander seeds
- 1 teaspoon cumin seeds
- a pinch of dried chilli flakes
- ½ teaspoon dried thyme
- 175 g (6 oz) thick white fish fillet, such as **pollock**
- low fat cooking spray
- 2 teaspoons extra light mayonnaise
- 2 teaspoons sweet chilli sauce
- salt and freshly ground black pepper

For the vegetable salad

- ½ small red **pepper**, sliced into thin strips
- 1 small **carrot**, peeled and sliced into ribbons
- 1 **spring onion**, shredded
- 1 teaspoon lime juice

The spice crust adds plenty of flavour to the fish with a minimum of effort. It's important to grill the fish spice side up at first since this is the side you'll see on the plate.

1 Grind the coriander seeds, cumin seeds and chilli flakes in a pestle and mortar to make a coarse powder, then stir in the thyme and season. Spoon the spice mixture over the top of the fish, pressing the spices into the fillet until you have a thick coating.

2 Heat the grill to high and line the grill pan with foil. Spray the foil and the fish with the cooking spray and grill spice side up for 3–4 minutes until slightly crisp. Using a fish slice or spatula, carefully turn and grill for another 2–3 minutes, depending on the thickness of the fillet, until cooked through.

3 Meanwhile, make the salad by combining the red pepper, carrot and spring onion in a serving dish. Pour the lime juice over and season to taste.

4 Mix together the mayonnaise and sweet chilli sauce and serve with the fish and salad.

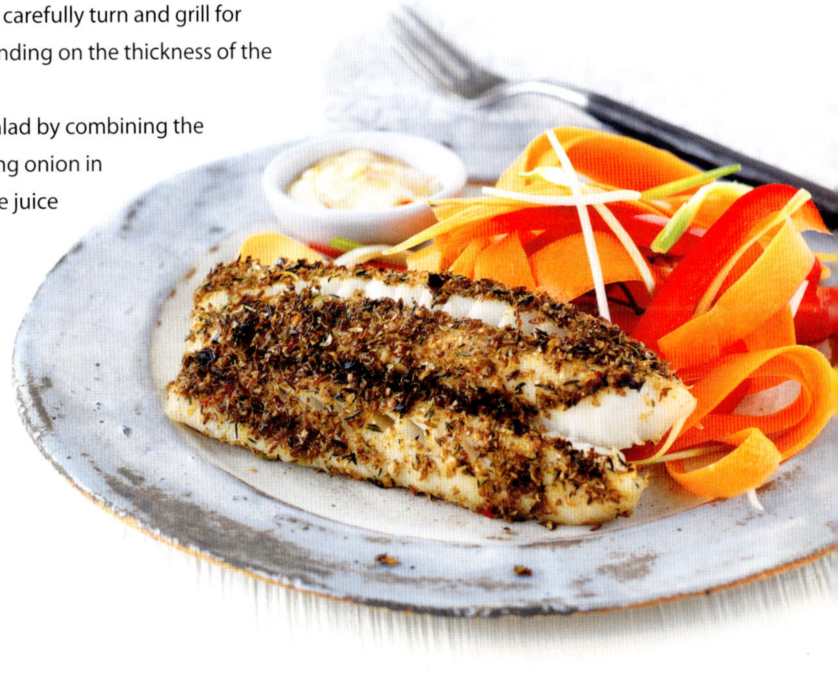

Roasted black bean tofu

7 *ProPoints* value

ProPoints **values per serving 7**
ProPoints **values per recipe 14**
Takes 40 mins + 30 mins marinating

V **Serves 2**

250 g (9 oz) **tofu**, patted dry using kitchen towel, and cut into cubes
low fat cooking spray
1 cm (½ inch) **fresh root ginger**, grated
1 **carrot**, peeled and cut diagonally
60 g (2 oz) **mange tout**, halved diagonally
60 g (2 oz) long stem **broccoli**, stems cut diagonally
1 **spring onion**, cut diagonally, to garnish

For the marinade
6 tablespoons black bean sauce
2 tablespoons dark soy sauce
1 tablespoon clear honey
½ teaspoon toasted sesame oil

The tofu is marinated in a combination of black bean sauce, honey and soy sauce then roasted to give it a golden coating. Serve with 50 g (1¾ oz) dried basmati rice per person, cooked according to the packet instructions, for an additional 5 ***ProPoints*** values per serving.

1 To make the marinade, mix together all the marinade ingredients in a shallow dish. Add the tofu and turn until it is all coated then leave to marinate for 30 minutes.

2 Preheat the oven to Gas Mark 5/190°C/fan oven 170°C. Spray a baking tray with the cooking spray and arrange the tofu on top, reserving the marinade. Roast for 20–25 minutes, turning halfway, until golden. Using your hands, squeeze the juice from the ginger into the leftover marinade and discard the remaining fibrous bits of ginger.

3 Meanwhile, heat a wok or non stick frying pan until hot. Spray with the cooking spray and stir fry the carrot, mange tout and broccoli for 2 minutes. Pour the marinade into the wok and stir fry for a minute until the vegetables are coated in the sauce.

4 Serve the vegetables topped with the tofu and the spring onion.

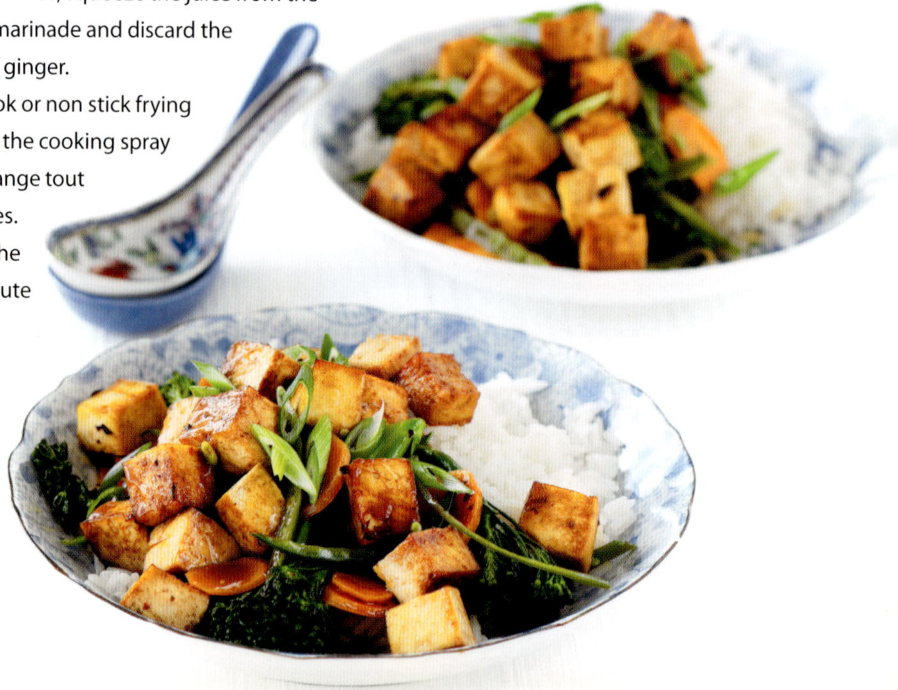

curries
and one pots

Who doesn't love a delicious curry or a comforting stew? This chapter is full of tasty ideas and with recipes for all occasions, you'll find plenty of inspiration here.

Beef dopiaza on page 48

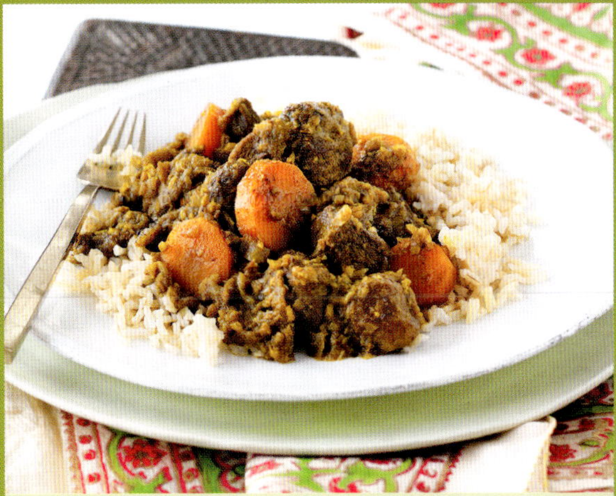

Pork kofta in red curry sauce

7 *ProPoints* value

***ProPoints* values per serving** 7
***ProPoints* values per recipe** 14
20 mins prep + 30 mins chilling,
20 mins cooking
Serves 2

200 g (7 oz) **extra lean pork mince**
2 large **spring onions**, chopped finely
3 large **garlic cloves**, crushed
2.5 cm (1 inch) **fresh root ginger**, grated
1 **egg**, lightly beaten
salt and freshly ground black pepper
1 tablespoon chopped **fresh coriander**, to garnish

For the red curry sauce

low fat cooking spray
1 small **onion**, chopped finely
1 tablespoon Thai red curry paste
100 ml (3½ fl oz) vegetable stock
100 ml (3½ fl oz) light coconut milk
2 tablespoons canned chopped **tomatoes**
1 tablespoon lime juice

Serve this curry with steamed **green beans** and 50 g (1¾ oz) dried **brown rice** per person, cooked according to the packet instructions, for an extra 5 ***ProPoints*** values per serving.

1 Mix together the mince, spring onions, two of the garlic cloves, half of the ginger and the egg in a bowl. Season, then using wet hands, form into eight balls, each about the size of a walnut. Arrange on a plate then cover and chill in the fridge for 30 minutes.

2 Meanwhile, to make the sauce, heat a large lidded saucepan, spray with the cooking spray and fry the onion for 5 minutes, stirring occasionally until softened. Add a little water if the onions start to stick. Add the remaining garlic and ginger then the red curry paste, and cook, stirring, for a minute.

3 Pour in the vegetable stock, coconut milk and chopped tomatoes and stir until combined. Bring to the boil then reduce to simmering point. Arrange the meatballs in the pan and spoon over the sauce. Partially cover the pan and simmer the meatballs for 15 minutes, turning occasionally, until cooked through.

4 Using a slotted spoon, remove the meatballs from the pan and arrange on two plates. Keep warm. Stir the lime juice into the sauce and then cook, uncovered, for another 5 minutes until thickened. Season to taste then spoon the sauce over the meatballs. Scatter with the coriander before serving.

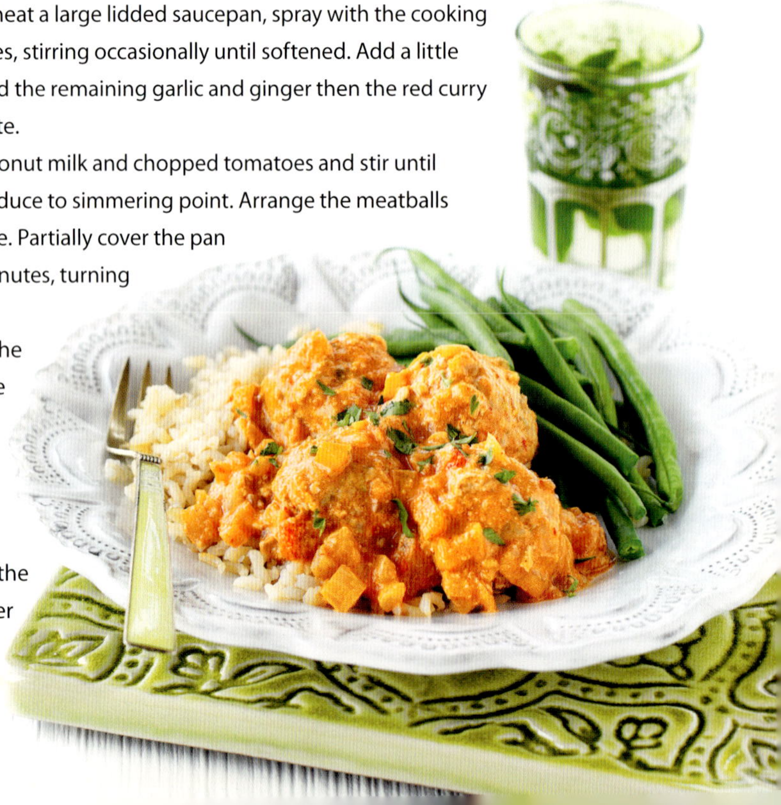

ProPoints values per serving 3
ProPoints values per recipe 6
Takes 35 mins

Serves 2

Thai green vegetable curry

- 75 g (2¾ oz) fine **green beans**, trimmed
- low fat cooking spray
- 250 g (9 oz) **aubergine**, sliced then quartered
- 2 tablespoons Thai green curry paste
- 300 ml (10 fl oz) vegetable stock
- 100 ml (3½ fl oz) light coconut milk
- 2.5 cm (1 inch) **fresh root ginger**, chopped finely
- 60 g (2 oz) **baby corn**
- 1 **courgette**, sliced diagonally
- 75 g (2¾ oz) chestnut **mushrooms**, halved
- 2 tablespoons chopped **fresh coriander**
- salt and freshly ground black pepper

Serve this fragrant and creamy coconut curry with 50 g (1¾ oz) dried jasmine rice per person, cooked according to the packet instructions, for an additional 5 ***ProPoints*** values per person.

1. Bring about 2.5 cm (1 inch) of water to the boil in a lidded pan. Put the green beans in a steamer basket and place it over the pan. Cover and steam for 5 minutes until almost cooked. Alternatively, bring a small amount of water to the boil and cook the beans for 5 minutes then drain. Refresh the beans under cold running water. Set aside.
2. Meanwhile, heat a large lidded non stick saucepan. Spray with the cooking spray and stir fry the aubergine for 7 minutes until softened. Add a little water if it starts to stick.
3. Spray the pan again with the cooking spray, add the curry paste and cook, stirring, for 1 minute. Pour in the stock and stir until combined then add the coconut milk, ginger, baby corn, courgette and mushrooms.
4. Bring to the boil, reduce the heat and simmer, partially covered, for 5–8 minutes until reduced and thickened. Season and stir in the green beans and a tablespoon of the coriander. Heat through and serve sprinkled with the remaining coriander and some black pepper.

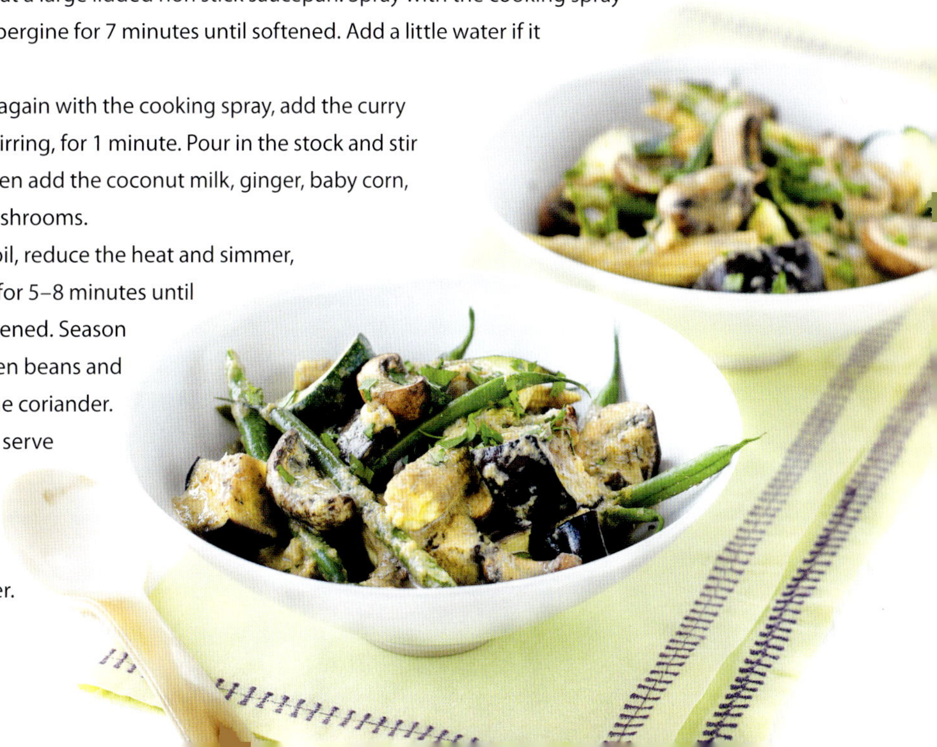

***ProPoints* values per serving** 8
***ProPoints* values per recipe** 16
20 mins prep, 1 hr cooking

Serves 2

- 200 g (7 oz) **onions**, chopped finely
- 4 cm (1½ inches) **fresh root ginger**, chopped
- 2 **garlic cloves**, chopped
- low fat cooking spray
- 1 teaspoon cumin seeds
- 250 g (9 oz) lean beef brisket, visible fat removed, and chopped into small cubes
- 2 teaspoons garam masala
- 1 teaspoon ground turmeric
- 1 large **carrot**, peeled and sliced thickly
- 200 ml (7 fl oz) vegetable stock
- salt and freshly ground black pepper

Beef dopiaza

8 *ProPoints* value

Serve this curry with 50 g (1¾ oz) dried **brown basmati rice** per person, cooked according to the packet instructions, for 5 additional ***ProPoints*** values per serving.

1 Place half of the onion, the ginger, garlic and 3 tablespoons of water in a food processor, or use a hand held blender, and whizz to make a paste.

2 Heat a medium size, lidded, non stick saucepan and spray with the cooking spray. Add the remaining onions, cover and cook for 5 minutes, stirring occasionally. Add the cumin seeds and beef. Cook for about 3 minutes until browned all over. Stir in the garam masala and turmeric.

3 Add the blended onion paste, carrot and stock and bring to the boil. Stir, then reduce the heat, cover and simmer for about 1 hour or until the beef is very tender. Add a little water if the sauce becomes too dry – the meat should be coated in a thick sauce. If the sauce is too thin at the end of the cooking time, remove the lid and simmer until reduced. Season to taste before serving.

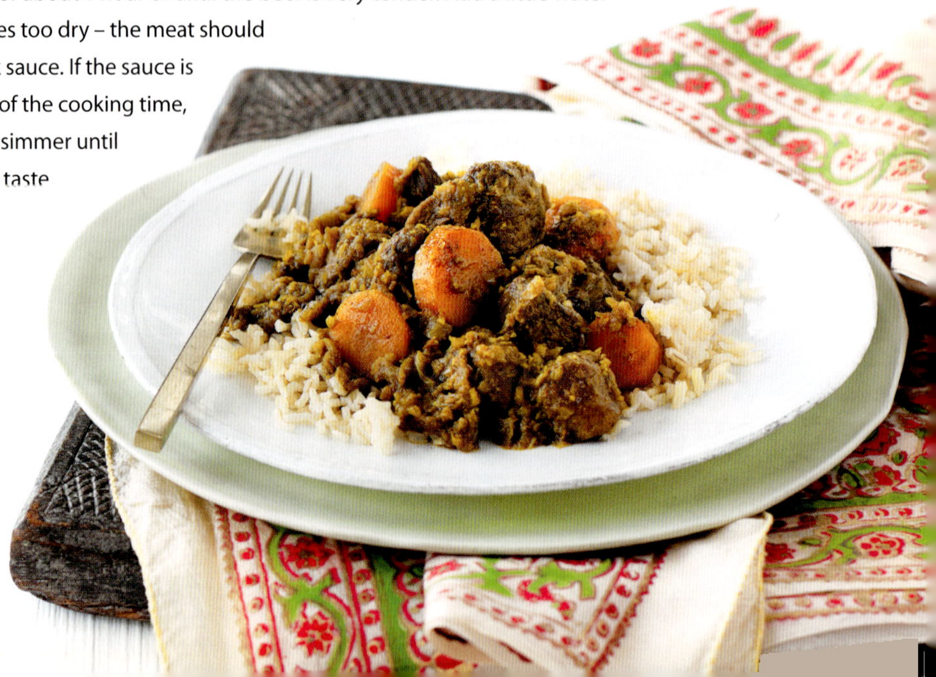

ProPoints values per recipe 11
Takes 30 mins

Serves 1

2 teaspoons tikka spice mix
100 g (3½ oz) lean boneless lamb leg steak, visible fat removed
low fat cooking spray
1 small **onion**, chopped
1 large **garlic clove**, chopped
1 teaspoon ground cumin
1 cm (½ inch) **fresh root ginger**, chopped finely
1 tablespoon Balti curry paste
200 g (7 oz) canned chopped **tomatoes**
50 g (1¾ oz) canned **chick peas**, drained and rinsed
75 g (2¾ oz) **spinach leaves**, tough stalks removed
2 teaspoons lime juice
salt and freshly ground black pepper

Lamb chana masala

11 *ProPoints* value

Curries don't have to take long to make as you'll see with this simple recipe. Serve with a plain poppadom for an additional 1 ***ProPoints*** value.

1. Rub the tikka spice mix all over the lamb. Season and then set aside.
2. Heat a lidded non stick saucepan and spray with the cooking spray. Add the onion, cover and cook for 5 minutes, stirring occasionally. Add the garlic, cumin and ginger then stir in the curry paste. Cook for a minute before you add the chopped tomatoes and chick peas.
3. Bring the tomato mixture up to the boil, then reduce the heat and simmer, partially covered, for 5 minutes. Stir in the spinach and lime juice, season, and cook for another 5 minutes.
4. While the curry is cooking, heat a lidded non stick frying pan. Spray the lamb with the cooking spray and cook for 2–3 minutes on each side, depending on the thickness of the lamb, until browned and cooked to your liking. Remove from the heat, cover and leave to rest for a few minutes.
5. Slice the lamb on the diagonal and serve on top of the curry.

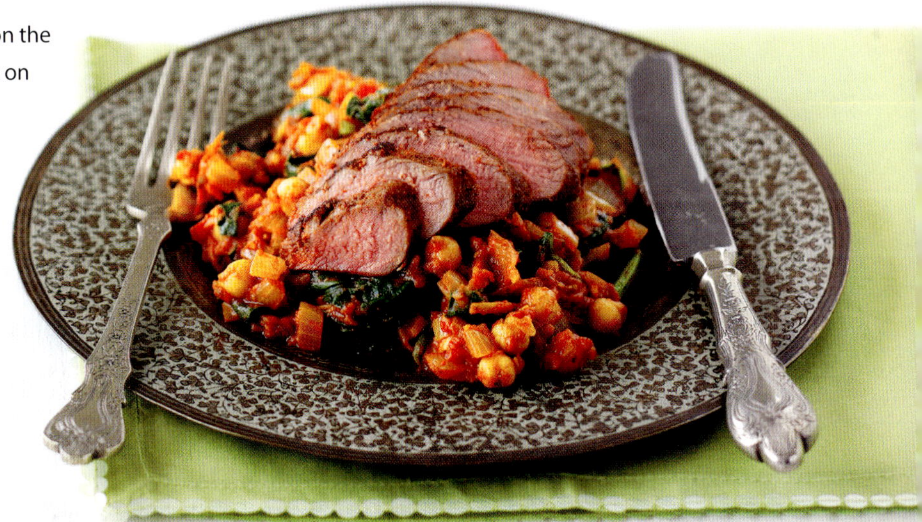

ProPoints values per serving 6
ProPoints values per recipe 23
20 mins prep, 25 mins cooking

Serves 4

- 4 cm (1½ inches) **fresh root ginger**, chopped
- 3 large **garlic cloves**, chopped
- 4 cardamom pods, lightly crushed with the flat blade of a knife
- low fat cooking spray
- 1 large **onion**, chopped finely
- 60 g (2 oz) chicken korma paste
- 1 teaspoon turmeric
- 200 g (7 oz) canned chopped **tomatoes**
- 200 g (7 oz) vegetable stock
- 550 g (1 lb 3 oz) **skinless boneless chicken breasts**, cut into large bite size pieces
- 12 cherry **tomatoes**, halved
- 4 tablespoons Weight Watchers reduced fat thick cream
- salt and freshly ground black pepper
- 4 lime wedges, to serve

Quick chicken korma

6 *ProPoints* value

With its deliciously mild and creamy sauce, korma is one of the most popular Indian curries and sure to appeal to the whole family. Serve with 50 g (1¾ oz) dried **brown basmati rice** per person, cooked according to the packet instructions, for an additional 5 ***ProPoints*** values per serving.

1 Place the ginger and garlic with 3 tablespoons of water in a food processor, or use a hand held blender, and whizz to a paste. Set aside.

2 Heat a large lidded saucepan. Add the cardamom pods and stir for 30 seconds then spray with the cooking spray and add the onion. Stir fry for 6 minutes until softened then add the korma paste, ginger paste mixture and turmeric.

3 Pour in the chopped tomatoes and stock then bring up to the boil. Reduce the heat to medium low, add the chicken and then simmer, partially covered, for 20 minutes, stirring occasionally.

4 Add the cherry tomatoes and cream then simmer for another 5 minutes until the sauce is reduced and thickened. Remove the cardamom pods. Season to taste and squeeze over the lime, to serve.

V Variation Instead of chicken, you could use 350 g (12 oz) **Quorn pieces** and 100 g (3½ oz) chestnut **mushrooms**, for 4 ***ProPoints*** values per serving. Add them in step 3 and cook for 10 minutes.

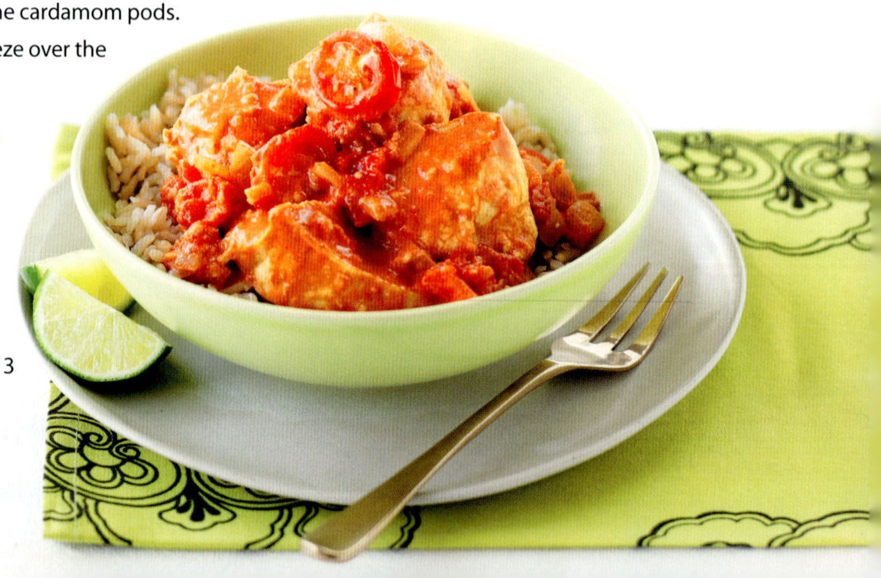

ProPoints values per recipe 7
10 mins prep, 20 mins cooking

Serves 1

3 tablespoons dark soy sauce
2 tablespoons Chinese cooking wine or dry sherry
1 star anise
1 cm (½ inch) **fresh root ginger,** sliced into matchsticks
1 clove
½ teaspoon grated orange zest
juice of ½ an orange
¼ teaspoon sugar
150 g (5½ oz) **skinless boneless chicken breast**

Red cooked chicken

7 *ProPoints* value

Star anise, soy sauce, orange and cloves add a fragrant oriental flavour and red colour to the chicken breast. Serve with steamed **pak choi** and 40 g (1½ oz) dried **brown basmati rice**, cooked according to the packet instructions, for an additional 4 ***ProPoints*** values.

1 Put the soy sauce, Chinese cooking wine or sherry, star anise, ginger, clove, orange zest and juice and sugar in a lidded saucepan and bring to the boil. Turn off the heat, cover and leave for 5 minutes to allow the flavours to infuse.

2 Add the chicken to the pan, spoon over the sauce and return to the boil. Reduce the heat and simmer, covered, for 15–20 minutes, turning the chicken halfway through and occasionally spooning over the sauce.

3 Remove the chicken from the sauce and slice thickly on the diagonal. Serve with a little of the sauce spooned over.

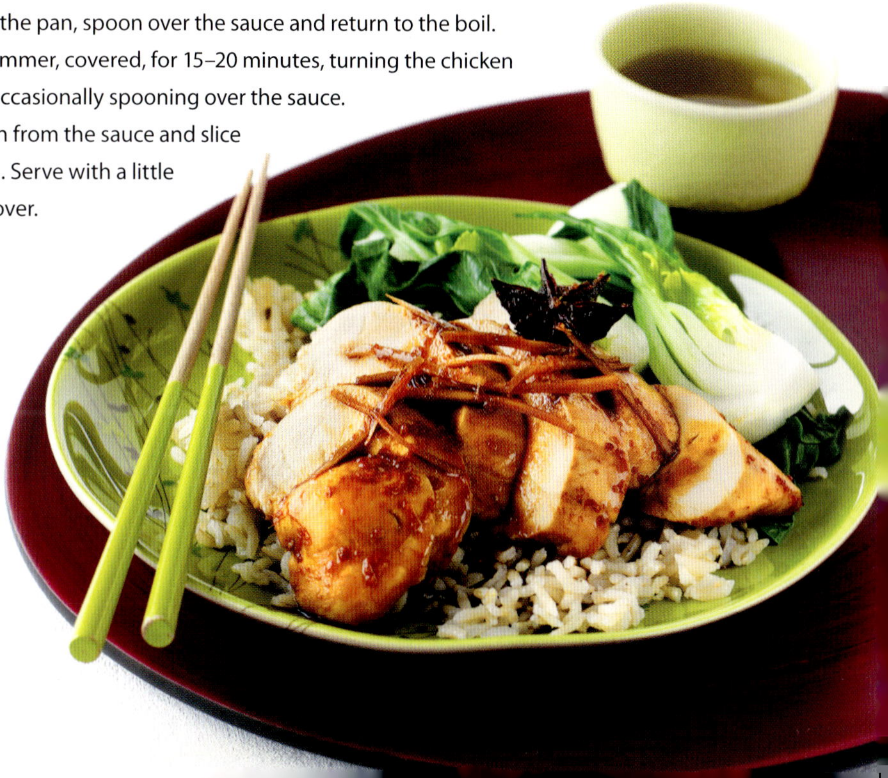

ProPoints values per serving 5
ProPoints values per recipe 20
Takes 45 mins

Serves 4

low fat cooking spray
1 **onion**, chopped finely
1 **corn on the cob**, kernels sliced off
1 red **pepper**, de-seeded and diced
1 **carrot**, peeled and halved lengthways, then sliced
2.5 cm (1 inch) **fresh root ginger**, grated finely
3 tablespoons Chinese cooking wine or dry sherry
1.2 litres (2 pints) fish or chicken stock
2 tablespoons light soy sauce
1 heaped tablespoon cornflour
450 g (1 lb) skinless white fish such as **whiting** or **pollock**, filleted and cut into large bite size chunks
150 g (5½ oz) cooked and peeled **prawns**, defrosted if frozen
2 tablespoons finely chopped **fresh coriander**
2 **spring onions**, sliced diagonally
freshly ground black pepper

Chinese seafood & corn broth

A delicious combination of fresh vegetables and seafood, this filling soup makes a perfect weekend lunch.

1 Heat a large, heavy bottomed, lidded saucepan. Spray with the cooking spray and cook the onion over a medium heat, covered, for 5 minutes, stirring occasionally, until softened, adding a little water if it starts to stick.

2 Add the corn, red pepper and carrot, cover, and cook for another 3 minutes, stirring occasionally. Add the ginger and pour in the Chinese cooking wine or sherry, which will bubble and hiss when added to the pan. Continue to cook for a minute until the wine has reduced.

3 Pour in the stock and soy sauce then bring to the boil over a medium heat. Mix the cornflour with a little cold water and add to the pan then stir well until combined. Reduce the heat and simmer for 10 minutes until thickened slightly.

4 Add the fish and gently simmer, stirring occasionally, for 4 minutes. Add the prawns and cook for a further minute until the fish is cooked. Season with black pepper to taste.

5 Divide the soup between four large shallow bowls, and sprinkle over the coriander and spring onions before serving.

Variation You could use 125 g (4½ oz) frozen or tinned **sweetcorn** in water instead of fresh. The ***ProPoints*** values will remain the same.

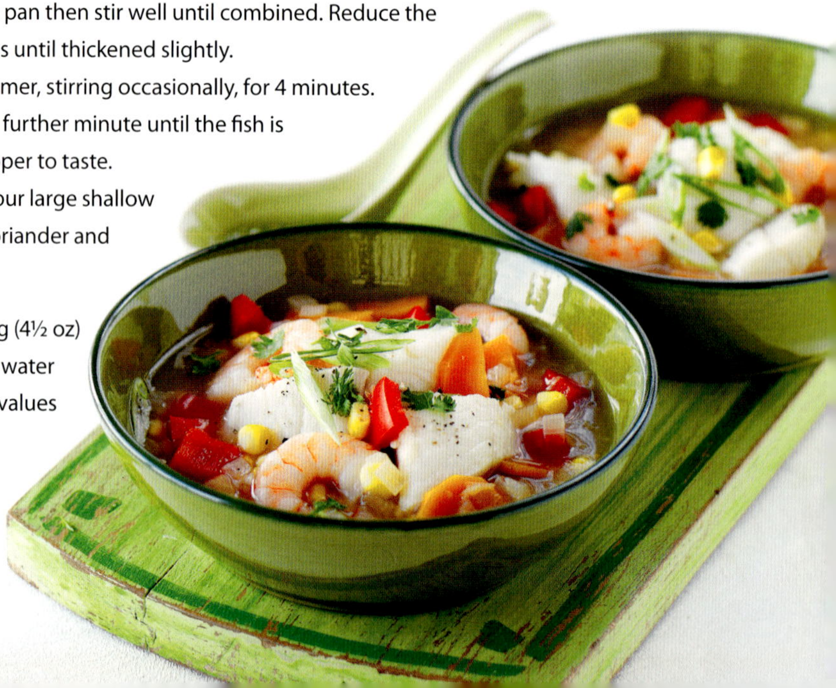

Mussels with lime & ginger

7 *ProPoints* value

ProPoints **values per serving 7**
ProPoints **values per recipe 14**
Takes 35 mins

Serves 2

- 1 kg (2 lb 4 oz) **mussels** in shells
- 2 **shallots**, chopped
- low fat cooking spray
- 1 **lemongrass stalk**, peeled and chopped finely
- 2 large **garlic cloves**, chopped
- 4 cm (1½ inches) **fresh root ginger**, chopped finely
- 2 dried kaffir lime leaves
- 4 tablespoons Chinese cooking wine or dry sherry
- 125 ml (4 fl oz) vegetable stock
- 1 heaped tablespoon Thai tom yam paste
- juice of ½ a lime
- 2 tablespoons chopped **fresh coriander**

Tom yam paste can vary in heat so use a little at first then add to taste.

1. Pull off any beards (the wiry strands that protrude from the shell) from the mussels. Scrape off any barnacles using a short, sturdy knife, then rinse well under cold running water. Discard any mussels with broken shells or those that remain open when tapped.
2. Heat a large lidded saucepan, add the shallots and spray them with the cooking spray. Fry the shallots, stirring, for 2 minutes. Add the lemongrass, garlic, ginger and kaffir lime leaves, then cook for another 30 seconds, adding a splash of water if it starts to stick.
3. Pour in the Chinese cooking wine or sherry and the stock and bring to the boil. Reduce the heat, stir in the tom yam paste and simmer for 2 minutes until the liquid has reduced slightly.
4. Add the mussels to the pan, cover with a tight fitting lid, and simmer over a medium heat, shaking the pan occasionally for about 4–5 minutes or until the mussel shells open. Discard any that remain closed.
5. Tip the mussels into a large colander placed over a bowl then cover to keep warm. Carefully pour the cooking liquid back into the pan, leaving behind any sediment in the bottom of the bowl. Stir in the lime juice and coriander and heat through. Divide the mussels between two bowls and pour the cooking liquid over before serving.

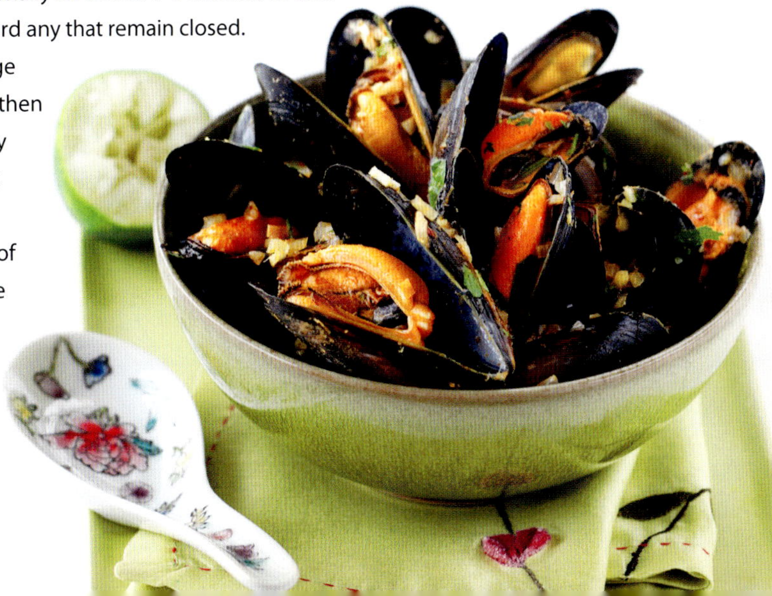

ProPoints **values per serving 4**
ProPoints **values per recipe 14**
20 mins prep, 25 mins cooking

Serves 4

low fat cooking spray
1 large onion, chopped
4 large carrots, peeled and sliced
1 large celery stick, sliced
125 g (4½ oz) dried split red lentils
2 bay leaves
2 cardamom pods, split
1 tablespoon garam masala
1 teaspoon ground turmeric
2 teaspoons ground cumin
1.2 litres (2 pints) vegetable stock
1 tablespoon lemon juice
4 tablespoons 0% fat Greek yogurt
salt and freshly ground black pepper

Spicy carrot & lentil soup

This thick vegetable and red lentil soup is lightly spiced with garam masala. Serve with a warm wholemeal chapatti each for an additional 4 ***ProPoints*** values per serving.

1 Heat a large, lidded, non stick saucepan. Spray with the cooking spray, add the onion and cook over a medium heat, covered, for 4 minutes until softened, adding a little water if they start to stick. Add the carrots and celery and cook, stirring occasionally, for another 2 minutes.

2 Stir in the lentils, bay leaves, cardamom and ground spices. Pour in the stock and bring to the boil then reduce the heat and simmer, partially covered, for 20–25 minutes until the lentils are soft.

3 Remove the bay leaves and cardamom pods and purée the soup using a hand held blender, or transfer to a food processor. Season to taste and stir in the lemon juice.

Serve topped with a spoonful of yogurt each.

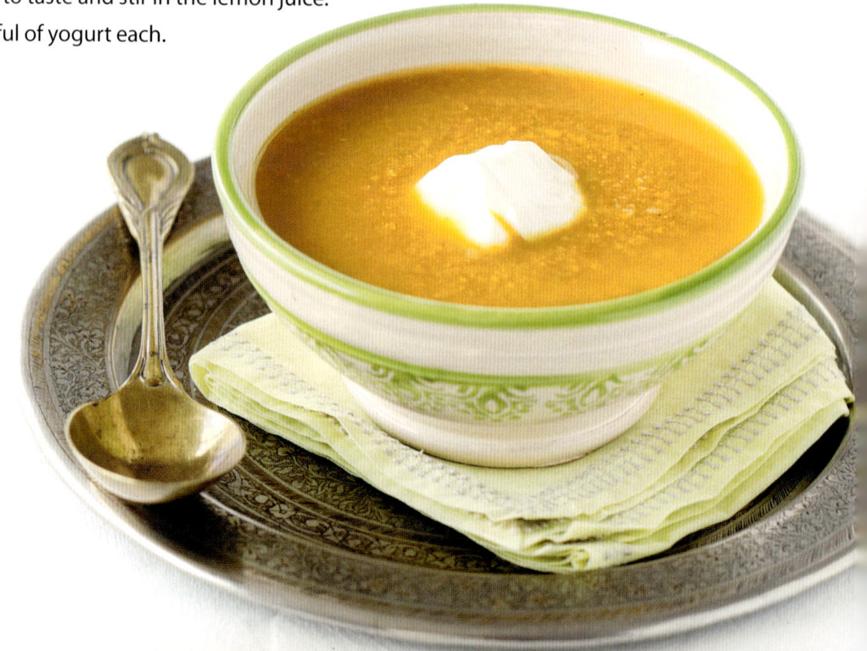

***ProPoints* values per serving** 8
***ProPoints* values per recipe** 33
25 mins prep, 1 hr 35 mins cooking

Serves 4

Oriental beef with butternut squash

- 500 g (1 lb 2 oz) lean beef brisket, visible fat removed, and diced
- low fat cooking spray
- 2 **onions**, sliced
- 1 star anise
- 1 teaspoon Chinese five spice
- 5 cm (2 inches) **fresh root ginger**, sliced finely
- 100 ml (3½ fl oz) fresh orange juice
- 5 tablespoons dark soy sauce
- 1 red **chilli**, de-seeded and chopped (optional)
- 450 g (1 lb) **butternut squash**, peeled, de-seeded and cut into large, bite size pieces
- salt and freshly ground black pepper

In this aromatic beef stew, the meat is cooked slowly in a sauce flavoured with orange juice, Chinese five spice and star anise.

1. Heat a large lidded casserole dish. Spray the beef with the cooking spray and add half of the meat to the pan, searing it until browned all over. Using a slotted spoon, remove the beef and set to one side. Repeat with the remaining beef.
2. Once all the beef has been seared and removed, put the onions in the pan, spray with the cooking spray, and cook over a medium heat for 4 minutes, stirring occasionally. Add the star anise, Chinese five spice and ginger then stir fry for a minute.
3. Pour in 400 ml (14 fl oz) water, the orange juice, soy sauce, and chilli, if using. Stir and then add the beef. Bring to the boil, then reduce the heat, cover, and simmer for 1 hour.
4. Add the squash and cook for 30 minutes, partially covered, or until the squash and beef are tender and the sauce is reduced and thickened. If the sauce is too thin, remove the lid, and cook for a few more minutes. Season to taste before serving.

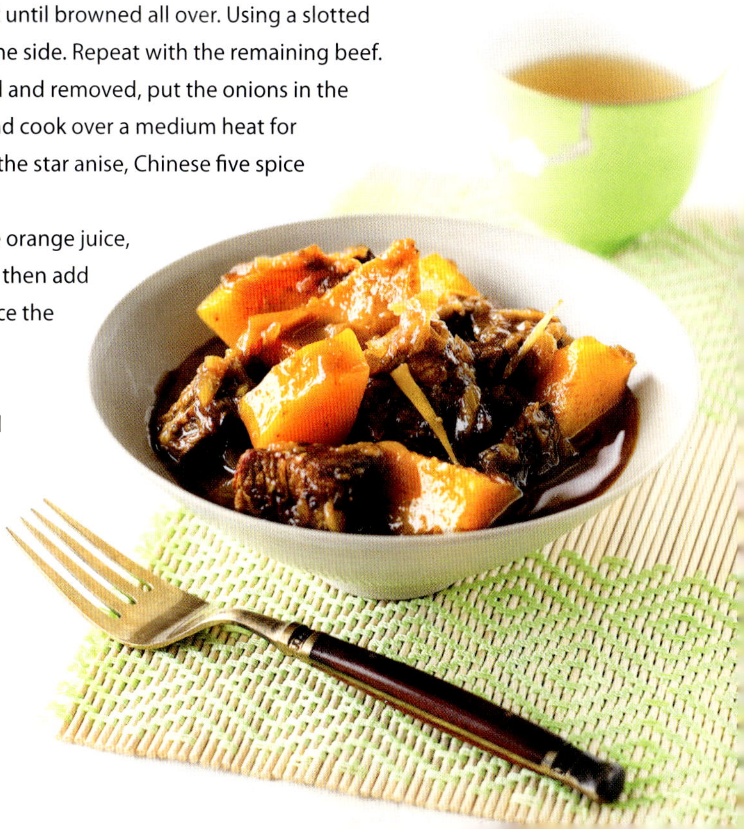

***ProPoints* values per serving** 7
***ProPoints* values per recipe** 29
20 mins prep + 1 hr marinating,
25 mins cooking
Serves 4

8 x 100 g (3½ oz) skinless **chicken drumsticks**
2 large **garlic cloves**, chopped roughly
2 tablespoons **fresh mint**
2 tablespoons tandoori spice mix
1 teaspoon ground turmeric
½ teaspoon chilli powder
juice of a small lemon
6 tablespoons **low fat natural yogurt**
low fat cooking spray
salt and freshly ground black pepper

For the onion salad

1 red **onion**, sliced thinly
6 **tomatoes**, de-seeded and diced
4 **radishes**, sliced into rounds
5 cm (2 inches) **cucumber**, quartered, de-seeded and diced
2 tablespoons lime juice

Tandoori chicken with onion salad

7 *ProPoints* value

The lightly spiced yogurt marinade helps to keep the chicken wonderfully moist and tender during cooking. Accompany with a warmed plain mini naan each for an extra 3 ***ProPoints*** values per serving.

1 Preheat the oven to Gas Mark 6/200°C/fan oven 180°C. Make two deep cuts on either side of each drumstick. Put the garlic, half of the mint, spices, lemon juice and yogurt in a blender or food processor or use a hand held blender and make a purée. Transfer to a shallow dish, season, add the chicken and spoon over the marinade. Cover and leave to marinate in the fridge for 1 hour.

2 Spray a baking tray with the cooking spray and add the chicken. Cook in the oven for 10 minutes then turn and spoon over some of the marinade. Cook for another 10–15 minutes until the chicken is cooked and there is no trace of pink inside and the outside is golden.

3 While the chicken is cooking, prepare the onion salad. Mix together the onion, tomatoes, radishes and cucumber. Squeeze the lime juice over, season and sprinkle with the remaining mint. Serve the salad with two drumsticks per person.

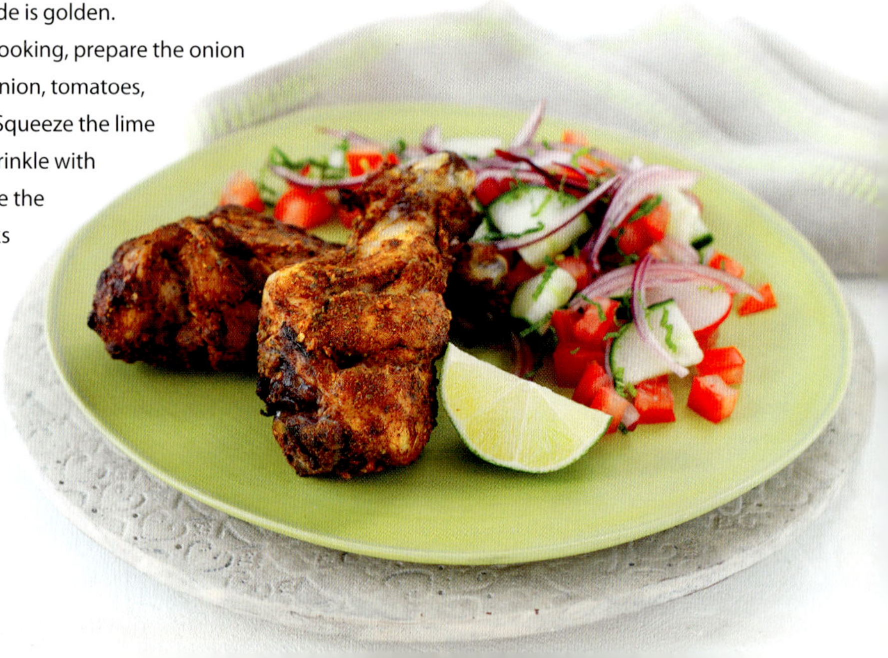

Shrikhand on page 63

desserts

These delicious desserts really hit the spot. Enjoy a creamy pudding, a refreshing sorbet or a warming and aromatic bowl of fruit poached in spices, for the perfect end to your meal.

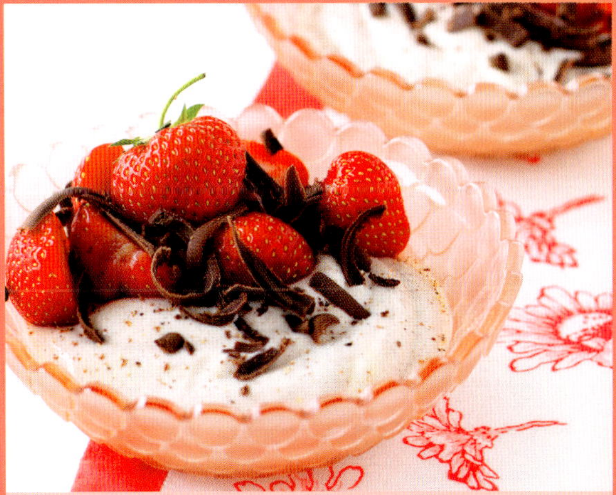

Fruit jelly with berries

***ProPoints* values per serving** **4**
***ProPoints* values per recipe** **14**
Takes 10 mins + 4 hrs setting

Serves 4

225 ml (8 fl oz) boiling water
135 g pack strawberry jelly, broken into cubes
150 ml (5 fl oz) light coconut milk
200 g (7 oz) mixed berries, such as **raspberries**, **strawberries** and **blueberries**, halved if large, to serve

The coconut milk and strawberry cleverly form two separate layers during setting to make an attractive dessert.

1 Put the boiling water into a measuring jug, add the cubes of jelly and stir well until dissolved. Pour in the coconut milk and make it up to 550 ml (19 fl oz) with cold water. Stir well until combined.

2 Pour the jelly into a four small clear glasses. Chill in the fridge for about 3–4 hours until set.

3 Serve with the berries scattered on top of the jelly.

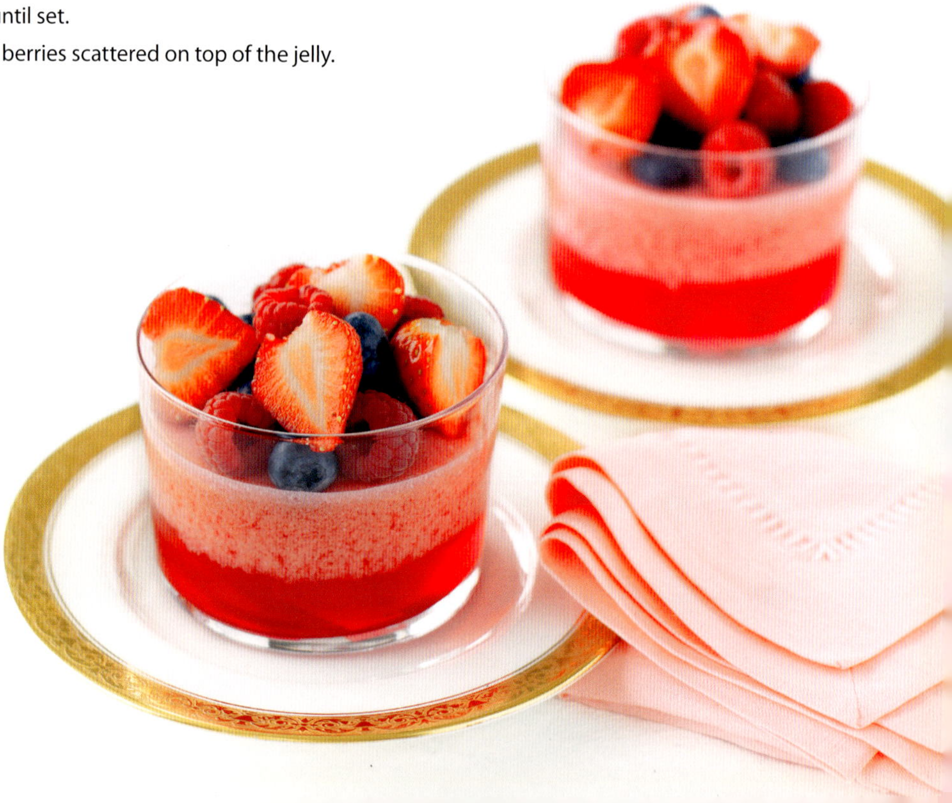

***ProPoints* values per serving** 7
***ProPoints* values per recipe** 28
Takes 15 mins + 30 mins resting

V ❄ pancakes only **Serves 4**

140 g (5 oz) self raising flour
1 tablespoon fructose or caster sugar
2 tablespoons unsweetened desiccated coconut
175 ml (6 fl oz) **skimmed milk**
1 **egg**, lightly beaten
low fat cooking spray
4 tablespoons **0% fat Greek yogurt**, to serve

For the caramelised bananas

2 large **bananas**, not too ripe, peeled and sliced thickly on the diagonal into ovals
zest of ½ an orange
4 tablespoons fresh orange juice
½ teaspoon ground cinnamon
2 tablespoons maple syrup

Coconut pancakes with caramelised bananas

7 *ProPoints* value

These American style pancakes are given a new twist with coconut and caramelised bananas.

1 Sift the flour and fructose or sugar into a mixing bowl, stir in the desiccated coconut then make a well in the centre. Pour in the milk then whisk in the egg to make a smooth batter. Set aside for 30 minutes.

2 Heat a large non stick frying pan and spray with the cooking spray. Using 40 ml (1½ fl oz) of the batter per pancake, cook 3–4 pancakes at a time. Cook for 1½–2 minutes per side until golden. Keep all the pancakes warm while you cook the caramelised bananas.

3 To make the caramelised bananas, spray the hot frying pan again with the cooking spray and place the bananas in the pan. Cook for 30 seconds or until slightly golden then turn over and cook for another 30 seconds.

4 Add the orange zest, orange juice, cinnamon and maple syrup and heat through for no more than a minute until the sauce is reduced and thickened. Place two pancakes on each serving plate and top with the caramelised bananas. Serve each with a spoonful of yogurt.

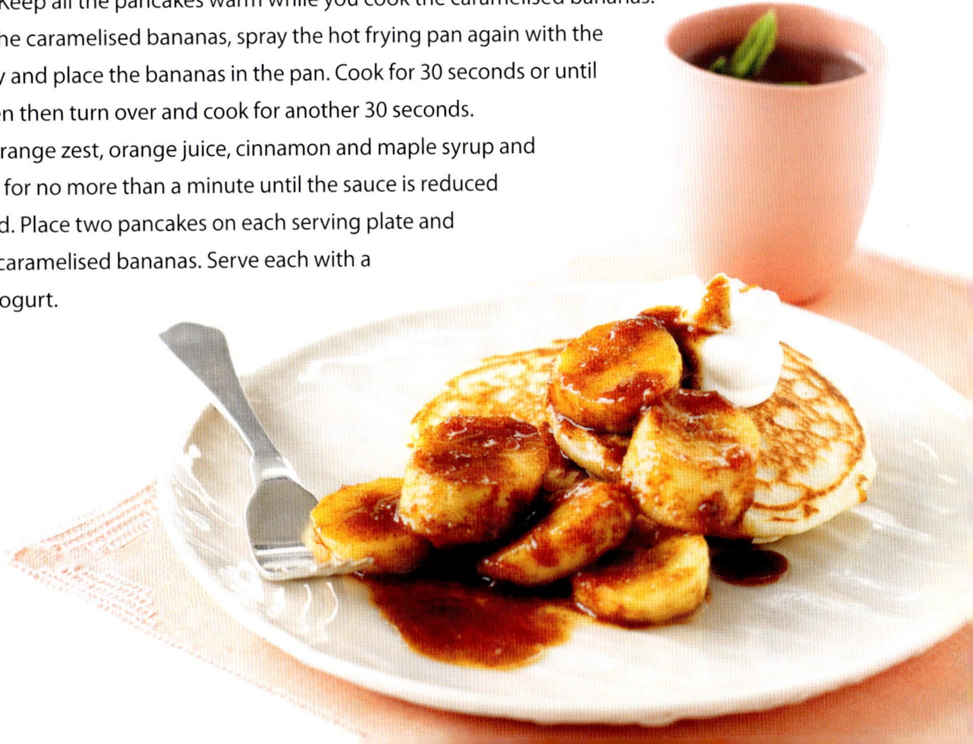

***ProPoints* values per serving** **1**
***ProPoints* values per recipe** **5**
Takes 10 mins + 5 hrs freezing
+ 20 mins softening
Serves 4

- 1 ripe **pineapple**, skin removed, cored, and cut into pieces, reserving any juice
- 5 cm (2 inches) **fresh root ginger**, grated
- 25 g (1 oz) stem ginger in syrup, drained and cut into small pieces
- 2 tablespoons fructose or caster sugar

Pineapple & ginger sorbet

This refreshing dessert makes the most of fresh pineapple, but is equally delicious using a 400 g can of **pineapple in natural juice**, drained, for the same ***ProPoints*** values.

1 Put the pineapple and any reserved juice in a food processor or blender and whizz to a coarse purée. Transfer to a mixing bowl. Using your hands, squeeze the ginger to extract the juice. Discard the remaining fibrous bits of ginger. Add the juice to the bowl with the stem ginger and fructose or sugar. Mix together.

2 Pour into a lidded freezerproof container. Freeze for 2 hours then stir with a fork to break down the ice crystals and return to the freezer for another 2–3 hours until frozen. Remove from the freezer 20 minutes before serving to allow the sorbet to soften.

Cook's tip If using fresh pineapple, make sure the fruit is perfectly ripe for the best flavour.

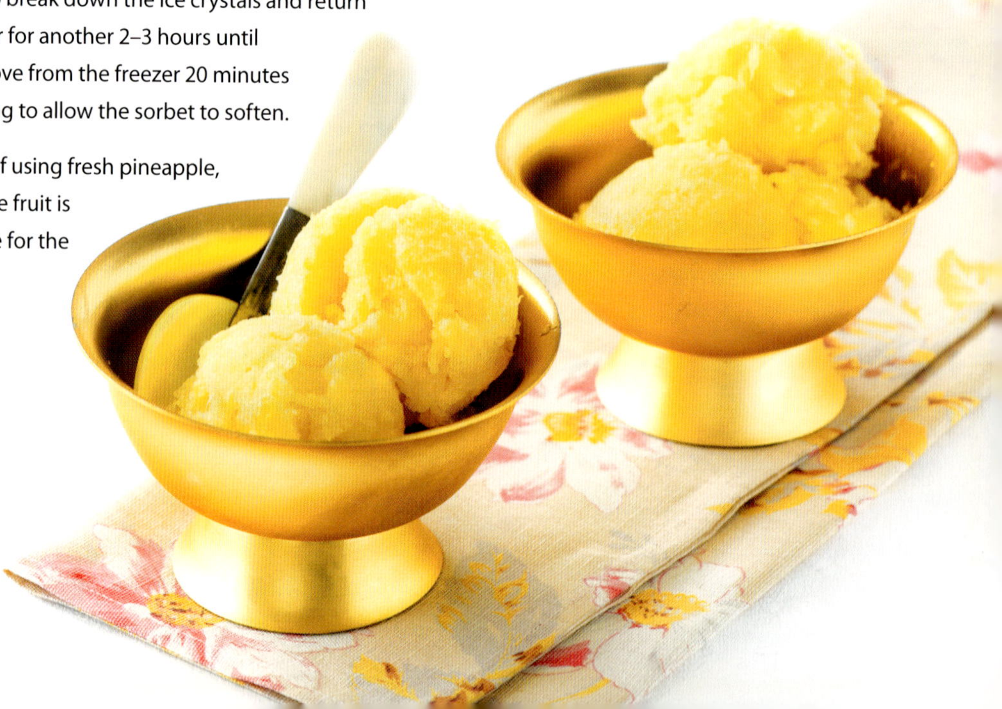

Mango kulfi

3 *ProPoints* value

***ProPoints* values per serving** 3
***ProPoints* values per recipe** 24
Takes 15 mins + 15 mins softening + 4 hrs freezing
Serves 8

1 large ripe mango
1 teaspoon vanilla extract
400 ml (14 fl oz) light evaporated milk
50 ml (2 fl oz) light condensed milk
low fat cooking spray
50 g (1¾ oz) unsalted shelled pistachios, chopped roughly

Kulfi is a classic Indian ice cream. This speedy version, flavoured with fresh mango, is just as delicious as the more time-consuming traditional method. If you don't want to serve it all at once, you could keep some in the freezer.

1. Using a vegetable peeler, remove the skin from the mango. Slice the fruit away from the stone, reserving a few thin slices to decorate. Put the remaining mango in a food processor, or use a hand blender, with the vanilla extract, evaporated milk, and condensed milk. Whizz until smooth and creamy.
2. Lightly spray eight 150 ml (5 fl oz) ramekins or dariole moulds with the cooking spray. Fill with the kulfi mixture. (You can also use a 1.2 litre/2 pint freezerproof container with a lid.) Freeze for 4 hours until frozen.
3. To remove the kulfi from the mould, remove from the freezer 15 minutes before serving, then run a knife around the sides. Turn upside down and give a little shake to release the ice cream from the mould on to a serving plate. You can also place the mould in a bowl of hot water for a few seconds to help to release the kulfi.
4. Serve one kulfi per person, sprinkled with the pistachios. Decorate with the reserved mango slices.

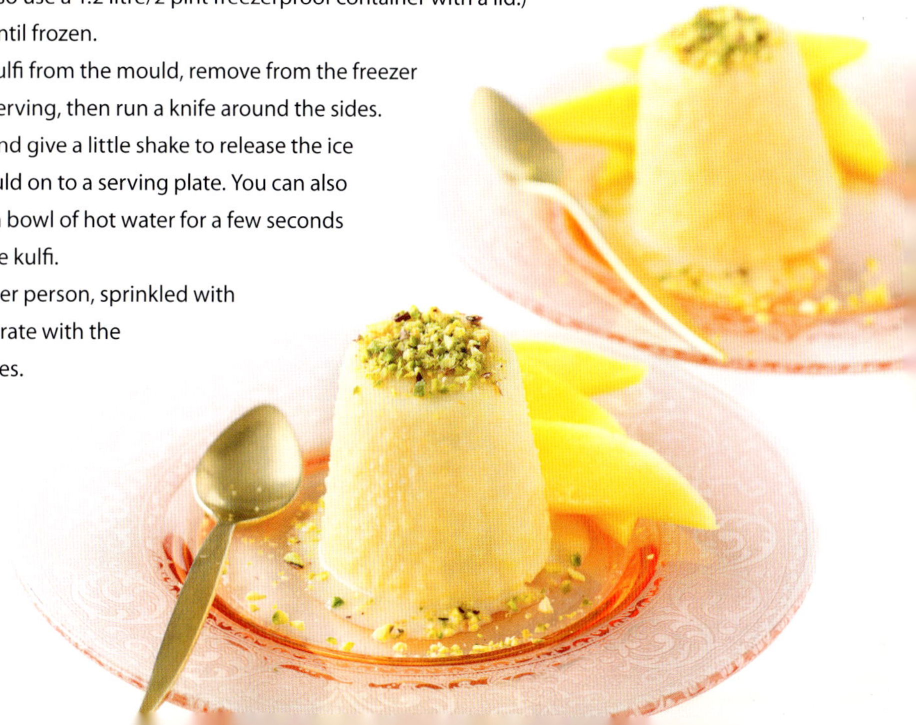

Mango lassi

***ProPoints* values per recipe** 8
Takes 5 mins

Serves 1

100 g (3½ oz) fresh **mango**, cut into chunks
5 tablespoons **low fat natural yogurt**
2 tablespoons **skimmed milk**
1 teaspoon fructose or caster sugar
15 g (½ oz) toasted flaked almonds, chopped roughly

Lusciously creamy and fruity, this traditional Indian drink makes a delicious light dessert or breakfast smoothie. For an indulgent twist, just before serving, add a 60 g (2 oz) scoop of reduced fat vanilla ice cream for an additional 2 ***ProPoints*** values for a delicious dessert.

1 Put the mango, yogurt, milk and fructose or sugar in a blender, or use a hand held blender, and blend until smooth and creamy. Pour into a tall glass, scatter over the almonds and stir in before serving.

Cook's tip Prepared fresh mango is available in the supermarkets.

Variation Why not freeze the mango mixture to make a fruity yogurt ice? Pour into a small freezerproof container with a lid then freeze until solid. Remove from the freezer 15 minutes before serving to allow it to soften.

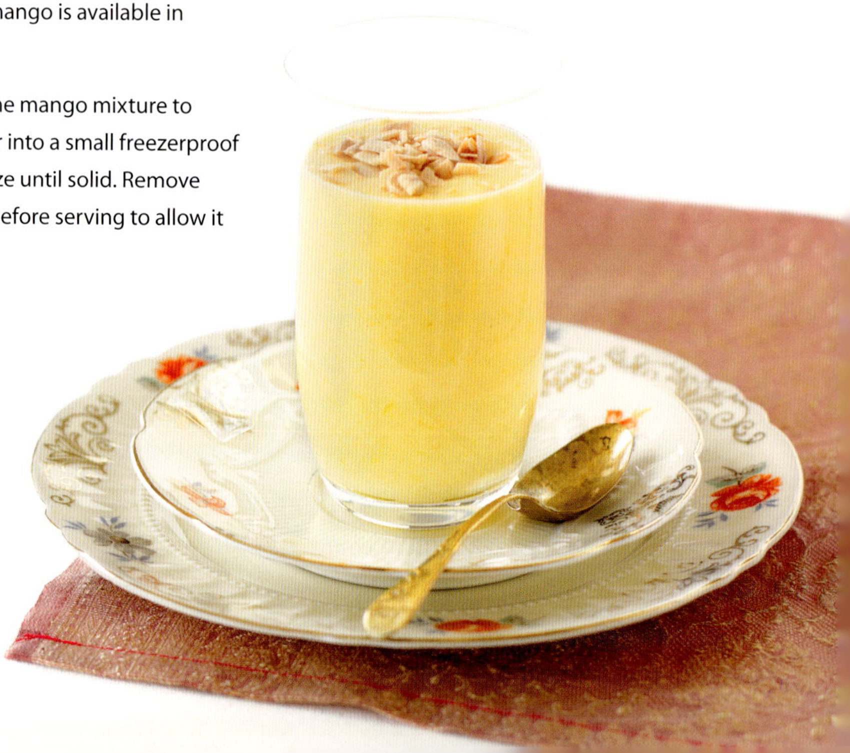

Shrikhand

ProPoints values per serving 4
ProPoints values per recipe 15
Takes 10 mins + 30 mins chilling

Serves 4

- 6 strands of saffron (optional)
- 2 x 150 g (5½ oz) pots 0% fat Greek yogurt
- 4 tablespoons Weight Watchers reduced fat thick cream
- 2 tablespoons golden caster sugar
- 1–2 teaspoons vanilla extract
- 1 teaspoon ground cinnamon
- 25 g (1 oz) dark chocolate
- ½–1 teaspoon ground nutmeg
- 200 g (7 oz) fresh strawberries, halved if large

This is the perfect dessert when you are looking for something sweet, creamy and indulgent but don't have much time on your hands. The saffron adds a distinctive yellow colour and flavour to this classic Indian dessert but can be left out, if preferred.

1 If using, soak the saffron in 1 tablespoon of hot water for 5 minutes to infuse. Put the yogurt, cream and sugar in a mixing bowl and whisk until thickened.

2 Gently stir in the vanilla, cinnamon and the saffron mixture, if using. Spoon into four small glasses or bowls. Chill for 30 minutes to firm up.

3 When ready to serve, using a vegetable peeler, slice the chocolate into curls. Sprinkle over the chocolate and nutmeg and top with the strawberries.

Cook's tip You can freeze this recipe to make a creamy yogurt ice. Pour into a freezerproof container with a lid then freeze until solid. Remove from the freezer 20 minutes before serving to allow it to soften.

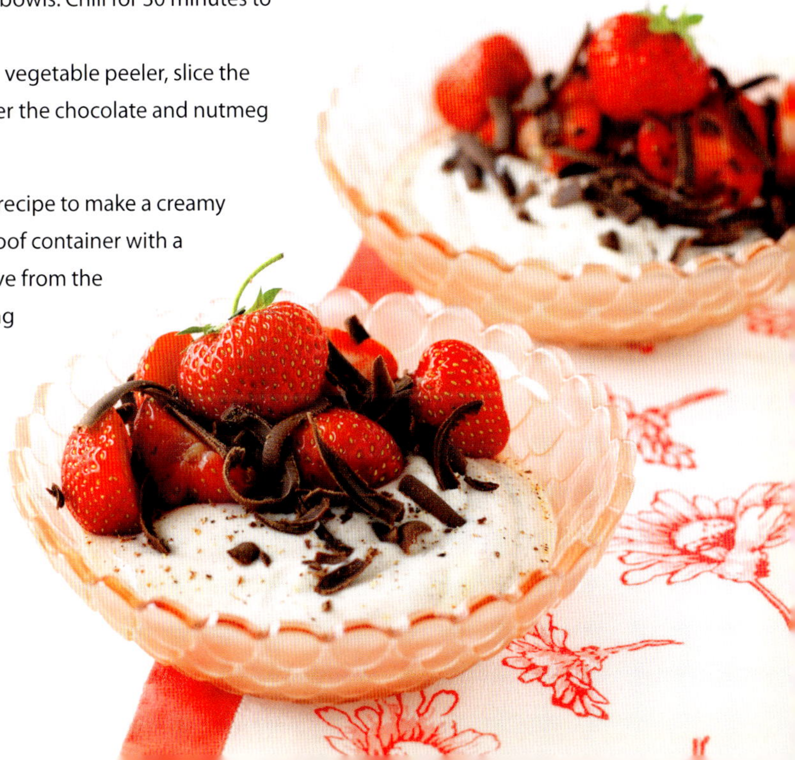

Apricots in cardamom syrup

8 *ProPoints* value

ProPoints **values per serving 8**
ProPoints **values per recipe 16**
5 mins prep, 20 mins cooking

V **Serves 2**

- 200 g (7 oz) dried apricots
- 3 cardamom pods, split
- 1 star anise
- 1 cinnamon stick
- 2 tablespoons clear honey
- 2 tablespoons Quark, to serve

Dried apricots become plump, soft and sweet when poached in a fragrant syrup. They're also delicious served for breakfast with natural yogurt.

1 Put the apricots in a lidded saucepan with 300 ml (10 fl oz) water and the cardamom, star anise, cinnamon and honey. Stir until combined then bring to boiling point.

2 Reduce the heat and simmer, partially covered, for 20 minutes until the apricots have softened and the sauce is syrupy. Remove the cardamom.

3 Serve the apricots in a bowl topped with a spoonful of Quark.

Cook's tip Look out for unsulphured apricots, which are dark golden in colour and have an almost toffee flavour.

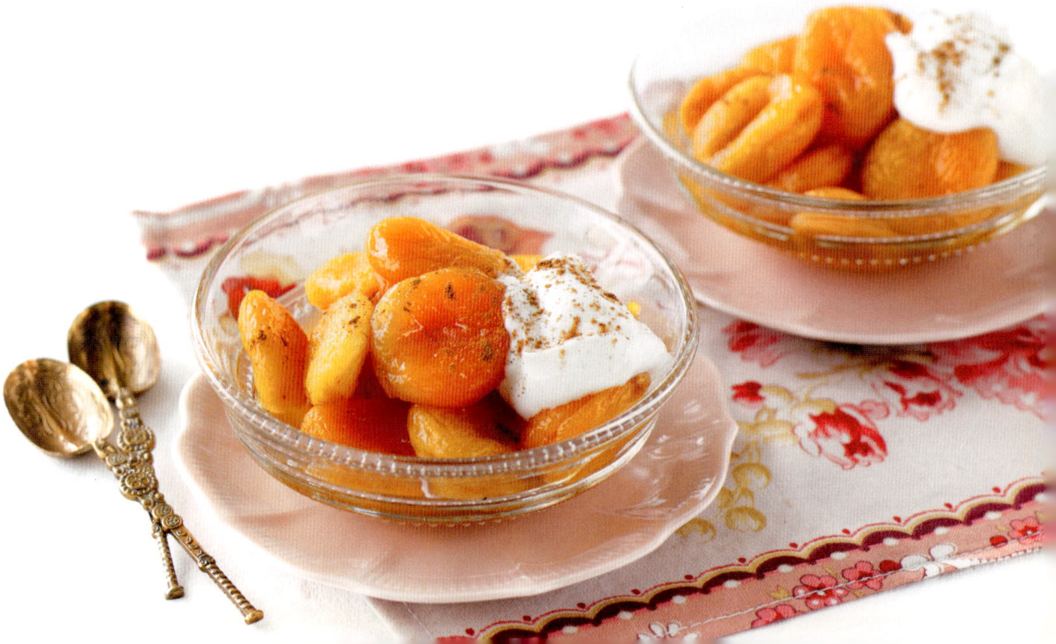

Oriental fruit salad

1 ProPoints value

***ProPoints* values per recipe** 1
Takes 10 mins

V **Serves 1**

4 **lychees**, peeled
125 g (4½ oz) **Charentais** or **Galia melon**, de-seeded and cubed
40 g (1½ oz) **blueberries**
2 tablespoons orange juice
1 teaspoon lime juice
1 **fresh mint sprig**, leaves removed
1 teaspoon grated lime zest
1 tablespoon **0% fat Greek yogurt**

The lime juice brings out the flavour of the fresh fruit, which comes with a citrus cream and is decorated with mint.

1. Put the lychees in a serving bowl with the melon and blueberries.
2. Pour over the orange and lime juice and scatter over the mint leaves.
3. Mix the lime zest into the yogurt and serve with the fruit salad.

Cook's tip You may prefer to stone the fresh lychees in step one. You could also use tinned lychees instead which are already stoned, for the same ***ProPoints*** values.

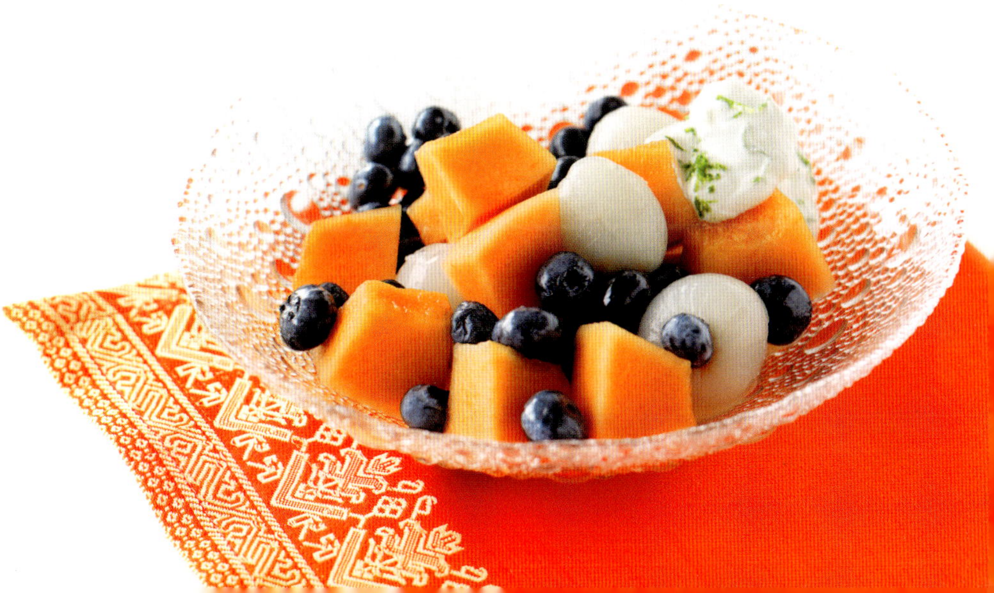

***ProPoints* values per serving** 8
***ProPoints* values per recipe** 15
10 mins prep, 35 mins cooking

Serves 2

75 g (2¾ oz) dried pudding rice
250 ml (9 fl oz) skimmed milk
2 cardamom pods, split
1 teaspoon ground cinnamon
2 tablespoons fructose or caster sugar
finely grated zest of ½ a small orange
3 tablespoons light coconut milk
½ teaspoon ground nutmeg
2 teaspoons toasted flaked almonds

Indian rice pudding

8 *ProPoints* value

This quick rice pudding is infused with cinnamon, orange and cardamom for a wonderful flavour and aroma.

1 Put the rice into a heavy based, lidded saucepan. Cover with 300 ml (10 fl oz) water. Bring to the boil, then reduce the heat and simmer, uncovered, for 15 minutes.

2 Pour the milk into the pan, then add the cardamom pods, cinnamon, fructose or sugar, and orange zest. Reduce the heat and simmer, partially covered, for 20 minutes, stirring regularly, or until the rice is tender. Stir in the coconut milk and heat through. Remove the cardamom pods.

3 Spoon the rice into small serving bowls, sprinkle with the nutmeg and top with the almonds.

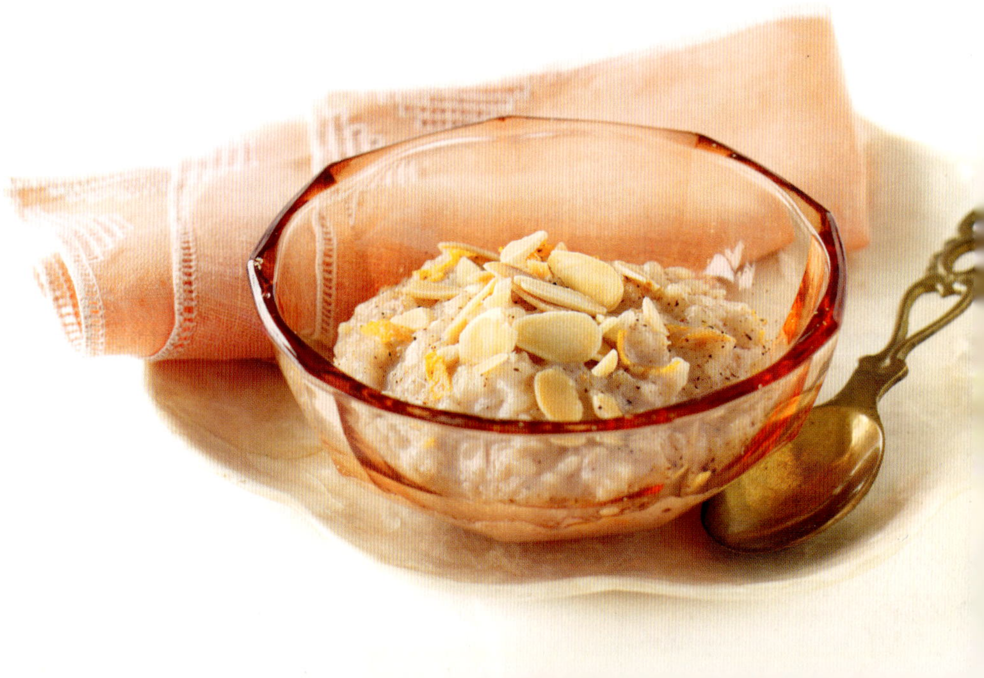

ProPoints values per serving 3
ProPoints values per recipe 13
Takes 20 mins

V Serves 4

- 1 **apple**, peeled, cored and cut into small dice
- 100 g (3½ oz) frozen **cherries**
- 2 **eggs**, separated
- 65 g (2¼ oz) caster sugar
- 100 ml (3½ fl oz) **skimmed milk**
- ½ teaspoon vanilla extract
- 2 teaspoons cornflour

Cherry blossom & snow

3 ProPoints value

In this pretty dessert, the fruit symbolises the first blossom of spring, while the meringue topping represents the snow that remains after the winter.

1 Put the apple, cherries and 2 tablespoons of water in a small lidded saucepan and simmer over a medium-low heat, partially covered and stirring occasionally for 9 minutes or until the fruit is cooked.

2 Meanwhile, put the egg yolks, 25 g (1 oz) of the sugar, the milk, vanilla, and cornflour in a heavy based saucepan and heat gently over a low heat, stirring constantly, until a thick and creamy custard is formed. This will take about 4–5 minutes.

3 Preheat the grill to high. Divide the fruit between four large 200 ml (7 fl oz) ramekins and spoon the custard on top.

4 In a clean, grease-free bowl, whisk the egg whites until they form soft peaks. Add half of the remaining sugar and whisk until combined then add the rest and continue whisking for a minute until they form firm, glossy peaks.

5 Spoon the meringue in peaks on top of the custard, spreading it out slightly. Place the ramekins on a baking tray and place them under the grill for about a minute until the peaks are slightly golden on top. Serve immediately or leave to cool.

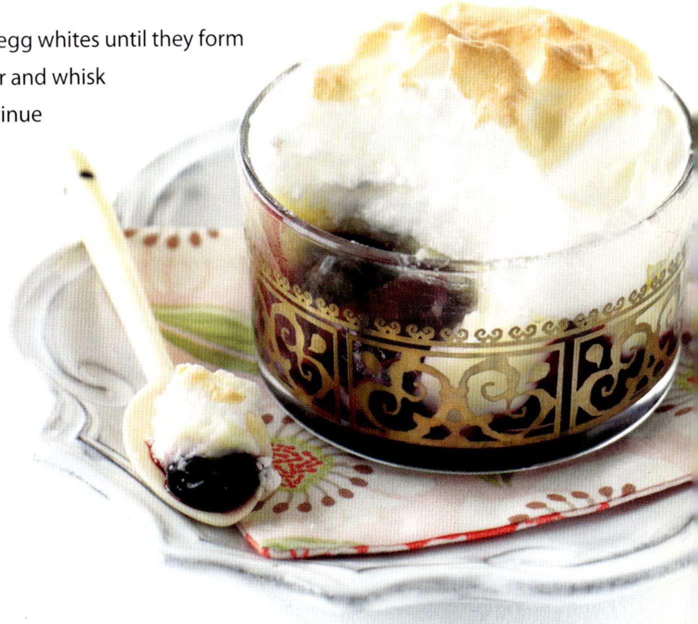

ProPoints values per serving 1
ProPoints values per recipe 2
15 mins prep, 30 mins cooking

Serves 2

2 slightly under-ripe pears, peeled and halved
1 teaspoon lemon juice
2 jasmine tea bags
4 thin slices fresh root ginger
1 cinnamon stick
1 tablespoon fructose or caster sugar
2 star anise

Jasmine tea & ginger pears

Pears are poached in jasmine tea and flavoured with aromatic cinnamon and star anise. Make sure the pears are slightly under-ripe to prevent them from becoming too soft when cooked. Serve with a spoonful of Weight Watchers thick cream for an additional 1 ***ProPoints*** value per serving.

1 Using a melon baller or teaspoon, scoop out the cores of the pears. Drizzle over the lemon juice to prevent them from browning.

2 Bring 850 ml (1½ pints) water up to the boil in a large, lidded, non stick frying pan. Reduce the heat and add the jasmine tea bags, stir and then simmer for 5 minutes.

3 Remove the tea bags from the pan, add the pears, ginger, cinnamon, fructose or caster sugar and star anise. Bring up to the boiling point.

4 Reduce the heat and simmer the pears for 15–20 minutes, partially covered, until tender then, using a slotted spoon, remove them from the pan. Increase the heat and cook for about 2–3 minutes, until the cooking liquid has reduced and thickened.

5 Serve two pear halves per person with the syrup spooned over the top. You may wish to serve the pears with the cinnamon stick and star anise since they look very attractive or you can remove them.

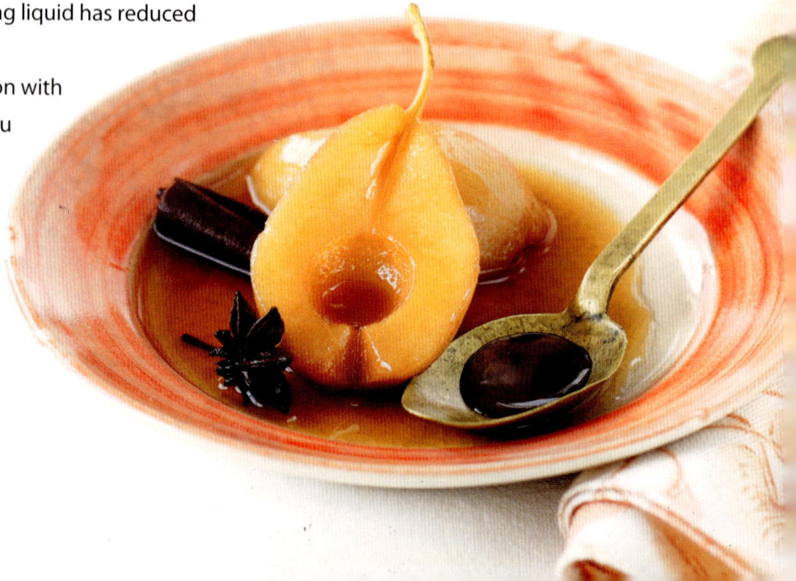